T0214725

Living-With Wisdom

Living-With Wisdom explores the way in which ancient Greek models of philosophy as an attempt to live 'the good life' can and should be realised through the practice of permaculture. Following the thought of Plato and Aristotle, the author places the achievement of wisdom and fulfilment at the centre of the good life, identifying these with the achievement of a complex admixture of virtues, which are dependent on an appreciation of goodness itself.

The book then examines the manner in which permaculture – or the practice of sustainable farming or ethical gardening – can provide us with the best opportunity to acquire this 'moral knowledge' through the close relationships we can have with other living beings and things. A study of the nature of wisdom and a means of 'living-with philosophy', *Living-With Wisdom: Permaculture and Symbiotic Ethics* reveals that it is by appreciating and sharing in the lives of other organisms that we engage with many dilemmas of life and death and have the opportunity to exercise the virtues.

As such, it will appeal to scholars of philosophy, social theory and anthrozoology with interests in virtue ethics, environmental ethics, animal ethics and human-animal relations.

Alexander Badman-King is an associate lecturer in the Department of Sociology, Philosophy and Anthropology at the University of Exeter, UK, where he is also a member of the Exeter Anthrozoology as Symbiotic Ethics working group.

Multispecies Encounters

Series editors:
Samantha Hurn is Associate Professor in Anthropology, Director of the Exeter Anthrozoology as Symbiotic Ethics (EASE) working group and Programme Director for the MA and PhD programmes in Anthrozoology at the University of Exeter, UK.
Chris Wilbert is Senior Lecturer in Tourism and Geography at the Lord Ashcroft International Business School at Anglia Ruskin University, UK.

Multispecies Encounters provides an interdisciplinary forum for the discussion, development and dissemination of research focused on encounters between members of different species. Re-evaluating our human relationships with other-than-human beings through an interrogation of the 'myth of human exceptionalism' which has structured (and limited) social thought for so long, the series presents work including multi-species ethnography, animal geographies and more-than-human approaches to research, in order not only better to understand the human condition, but also to situate us holistically, as human animals, within the global ecosystems we share with countless other living beings.

As such, the series expresses a commitment to the importance of giving balanced consideration to the experiences of all social actors involved in any given social interaction, with work advancing our theoretical knowledge and understanding of multi-species encounters and, where possible, exploring analytical frameworks which include ways or kinds of 'being' other than the human.

Other titles in the series:

Blogging Wildlife: The Perception of Animals by Hikers on the Appalachian Trail
Kate Marx

Totemism and Human-Animal Relations in West Africa
Sharon Merz

The full list of titles for this series can be found here: https://www.routledge.com/Multispecies-Encounters/book-series/ASHSER1436

Living-With Wisdom
Permaculture and Symbiotic Ethics

Alexander Badman-King

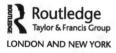

Routledge
Taylor & Francis Group

LONDON AND NEW YORK

First published 2021
by Routledge
2 Park Square, Milton Park, Abingdon, Oxon OX14 4RN

and by Routledge
605 Third Avenue, New York, NY 10158

Routledge is an imprint of the Taylor & Francis Group, an informa business

British Library Cataloguing-in-Publication Data
A catalogue record for this book is available from the British Library

Library of Congress Cataloging-in-Publication Data
A catalog record has been requested for this book

ISBN: 9780367406035 (hbk)
ISBN: 9780367695835 (pbk)
ISBN: 9780429357008 (ebk)

Typeset in Times New Roman
by KnowledgeWorks Global Ltd.

For MN, for being a good friend, a fellow philosopher, and making this and so many other things possible.

Contents

Acknowledgements

All of the philosophers whom it has been my privilege to know and learn from must be thanked here but I owe particular gratitude to Michael Hauskeller, who has been a source of guidance and inspiration throughout the process of writing this book. True philosophers are rarer than one might hope, and Michael is certainly one of them.

1 Moral knowledge ('wisdom') as the purpose of philosophy and life

What a Piece of Work is a Man?

(Shakespeare, *Hamlet*, 2.2)

ἐθος ανθροποι δαιμον.

(Heraclytus, *DK119*[1])

What is important? How do we find out what's important? And, once we know what's important how do we act in accordance with it?

These are the questions this book seeks to ask and, as much as I have been able, to answer.

There is a suggestion here, and it is not original to me, that it is more or less possible to live well and that doing so is the thing with which we humans should, first and foremost, be concerned. Discovering what is important and living in accordance with that discovery is the means by which we can live more or less well.

The suggestion which is more original to this book is that a very good way to discover what is important and to live in accordance with that discovery is to live with other living things. The way to learn how to live well is to grow plants, to care for animals, to breathe deep the good green things of this world, to perceive their value and to attend to that value.

But understanding importance, understanding value and one's own relationship with value, demands particular philosophical work. Even before we can introduce the idea of living with other living things as an effective means of discovering how to live well, we must first clarify the nature of value, the nature of moral knowledge and the nature of the means by which any such knowledge might be gained. That such things are even possible is, alas, far from ubiquitously accepted, either amongst scholars or those less familiar with the academic arguments around such topics.

The arguments and explorations of this book are conducted from and with a quite 'strong' form of moral realism, which is to say that the ideas expressed here (the answers to the questions) involve the suggestion that good and bad, right and wrong, are *real*, and that moral facts are possible.

This realism does itself require some justification and that too will comprise a notable chunk of the discussion here.

Similarly, when it comes to what is meant by 'living-with' and how one can acquire moral knowledge by this 'living-with', some significant explanation is called for. Ultimately, I will try to describe a method of ethical investigation which is largely inspired by (perhaps identical to) anthropological traditions of participant – observation, and how this method is (or should be) viewed as synonymous with philosophy when either of them is done the right way.

In the end, this book is itself an effort in trying to live well, it is an attempt on my part to live well, to help myself to live a slightly better life and, I hope, to help others to live well. It is a plea, however gentle or convoluted, for the reader to take the time, to make the effort, to pause and appreciate the fullness of truth and values that are readily apparent in the lives of all living things.

I call all of this 'philosophy', I also call it 'symbiotic ethics', they are, I think, the same thing. Anyone with any background in academic philosophy should also be told at this point that despite the many unorthodox departures which this book makes from usual philosophical processes of any tradition, it does, on the whole, belong to a tradition of English speaking philosophy, and particularly English speaking ethics. In many ways, the following arguments and explorations do not diverge dramatically from existing traditions of English ethics and, even more specifically, from a kind of philosophy which found its apogee in the 'ordinary language' and Oxbridge orientated conversations of the early and mid-20th century. Wittgenstein and Iris Murdoch are of particular importance, but that broader tradition of philosophy, its lucidity, openness and honesty, is something from which this book emerges and to which it aspires.

There's undoubtedly aesthetic conjunction between this peculiarly English tradition of philosophy, redolent of limestone common rooms and the kinds of gardening in which this book sets as its source of ethical inspiration. I hope that such aesthetic conjunction does not raise too much suspicion, too much incredulity that what follows could possibly represent a serious philosophical discussion. As Chapter 5 discusses, the aesthetics of both how we live and how our conversations unfold are far from irrelevant to how we should judge them, and any odour you find here of heavy bookcases and damp seedlings is not unintentional.

The terminology I have used to discuss gardens and gardening is something which is discussed in following chapters, but it is worth noting at the outset that 'permaculture' is only one of several possible terms which might be used. The most important thing to understand at this point is that the kind of gardening, agriculture or other living-with-the-land which I am discussing here is not primarily ornamental; it is more about growing food than flowers. There may be some people for whom the suggestion that permaculture and philosophy can be thought of as very closely connected or even identical is a perfectly natural suggestion, for others it may seem quite surreal, I hope my discussion here invites both into new and compelling ways of thinking about the world and our place in it.

Doing well

It is not a particularly novel suggestion that philosophy is something other (and more) than that which is done in classrooms and within the obscure lines of esoteric papers passed between mysterious academic cults. Within academic philosophy, there is a recognisable movement towards (or back to) a view of philosophy which considers it to be not a distinct pursuit so much as a 'way of life' (Hadot 1987, pp. 80–144).

The question is imagined as one of Socrates' making, or at least he is frequently viewed as the founder of western moral philosophy. How *should* we be? Who *should* we be? What *should* we do? Socrates asked questions about life rather than just about the substances and principles governing the world.[2] The *'we'* here is also important in a revival of ancient ethics. Even Socrates', in all his mischief, wasn't seeking to sever the individual entirely from his community. This was a world dominated by the identities and duties tied to the city-state, and any question about how life should be lived was inherently bound to the idea of collective duty.[3] The question then becomes not so much one of the individual duties and responsibilities (though these are still important) as one of *what it is to be a good human*. What are the qualities and activities which characterise a *flourishing* human life?

'Flourishing' is a popular term in 'philosophy as a way of life', it is an attempt, in part, to grapple with the Greek concept of εὐδαιμονία. Martha Nussbaum has been instrumental in this translation of εὐδαιμονία. In her 'Therapy of Desire', Nussbaum explains that the more traditional translation of 'happiness' 'is misleading, since it misses the emphasis on activity, and on completeness of life' (Nussbaum 1994, p. 15).[4] Yet 'happiness' does convey the sense in which εὐδαιμονία is considered as an end goal by the philosophers who employ it in their ethical discussions.[5] One can well imagine that happiness (as opposed to material wealth or power) would be viewed as a plausible and even laudable life goal by many people today. The revival of ancient Greek philosophy explicitly seeks to distance itself from the sort of inclination which might lead to this sort of individualistic, hedonic and static vision of purpose. 'Flourishing' speaks of potential and as such takes on the paternalistic tones of unfulfilled potential, languishing in supposed happiness. This is not a purpose to be arrived at through personal adventure and preference, or even cultural tradition, it is grander still, it is *Human*. Apart from this anti-hedonic mood, however, it is the emphasis on *activity* which Nussbaum highlights which has been crucial to the formation of philosophy as a way of life.

As opposed to other academic fields which take ancient Greek sources as intellectual points of interest and argumentative support, philosophy as a way of life takes the very model of ancient philosophy as an activity to be emulated. Against trends of specialisation and professionalisation in academia, it sets practical engagement, emersion and self-improvement as its mode of conduct. Pierre Hadot (whose work *Philosophy as a Way of Life* is the seminal text of this revival) sets forth an understanding of ancient ethics predicated upon an idea of philosophy as itself being a call to a particular ethical code closely allied to the pursuit of εὐδαιμονία (Hadot 1987, p. 102).

A translation of εὐδαιμονία as 'happiness' might allow for an academic integration of ancient ethics into a more modern scheme of liberal hedonism whereby the professional philosophers do philosophy because they enjoy it or because it affords them opportunity for other enjoyment. εὐδαιμονία as a more complex notion, however, introduces an unavoidable dissonance between profession and that which is professed.

εὐδαιμονία might literally be translated as well-spirit, and this may partly be to blame for the standard translation of 'happiness', it translates neatly as a noun concerned with psychological ease. If, though, a participle were allowed for, then 'flourishing' permits a far richer sense of the personal participation necessary to realise this condition. It is something which must be achieved not as a prize but as an activity. What 'flourishing' can lack, however, though it carries a sense of paternalism, is an explicitly moral sense. As Hadot emphasises, εὐδαιμονία is a complex idea which from its earliest records is not used in a univocal way but as part of a wider discussion of virtue and desired ends (*Ibid.*, pp. 264–269). σοφία (wisdom), ἀταραξια (peace of mind), ἀυταρκεια (inner freedom) and ἀρετή (virtue), all converge in these ancient discussions of life, ultimate meaning and our escape from suffering. Even the Epicureans, who diverged significantly from the Stoics in suggesting that pleasure does indeed take a central role in this mission, speak in normative and prescriptive ways about these goals. A challenge for philosophy as a way of life as a field, not just of academic study but of what might be called 'alternative therapy',[6] is to negotiate this normative character of ancient ethical discourse. This discussion seeks to explore in greater detail the moral dimensions of understanding philosophy as a way of life. What sort of way of life is this and what recommends it above other ways?

'Doing-well', as a translation of εὐδαιμονία, might capture that same sense of participation as flourishing and also carry a more explicit sense of moral orientation (as well as being a close to literal translation). If it were necessary to use a translation then this might suffice for the purposes of this discussion, but Nussbaum's preference for leaving the term in Greek seems a safer bet. When an idea is complex in a unique and interesting way, it forgives unique terminology.

A way of life for all?

It is telling that Pierre Hadot speaks explicitly of 'exercise spirituels' and couches the ancient practice of philosophy in this kind of religious language (Hadot 1987, pp. 264–269). Indeed, Hadot makes no bones about the continuity he perceives between ancient Helenistic ethical practices and the understanding of ethics many of us have inherited through Christianity.[7] Nor should we expect him to do otherwise, such musings are surely the raison d'etre of a chair of Hellenistic and Christian philosophy, and yet there are questions we may still ask. Chief amongst these questions is that as to whether the kind of 'spiritual' way of life being recommended is in fact the best, or even a good, way of life.

In what follows, no dissimulation shall be made in regards to the somewhat political, anti-intellectualist impetus behind this enquiry into the goodness of this Hellenistic ethics. Indeed, it is suggested that, in common with Aristotle's proposed ethical methodology,

> In matters of emotion and of action, words are less convincing than deeds; when therefore our theories are at variance with palpable facts, they provoke contempt, and involve the truth in their own discredit... Hence it appears that true theories are the most valuable for conduct as well as for science; harmonising with the facts, they carry conviction, and so encourage those who understand them to guide their lives by them.
>
> (Aristotle 335–323 BC § X,i (1172ᵃ34–1172ᵇ7)[8]

So let us be wary of ethics which, at times, encourages an almost ascetic detachment from day-to-day toil, which values above all else the activities of a contemplative mind and least of all those of physical work and bodily enjoyment, and let us be particularly wary of this for it having been recommended by scholars and priests. Aristotle is himself not insensitive to the possibilities of misconstruing his own ethics into one which demands the prerequisite of abundant good fortune and states that 'private citizens do not seem to be less but *more* given to doing virtuous actions than princes and potentates. It is sufficient then if moderate resources are forthcoming; for a life of virtuous activity will be essentially a happy life' (*Ibid.*, X, viii, x).

Iris Murdoch echoes this vein of concern in her own analysis of ancient ethics when she claims that 'it must be possible to do justice to both Socrates and the virtuous peasant' (Murdoch 1970, p. 2). And, whilst I might express this thought differently, I agree, it must. Indeed, the tension here lies just at that confluence of Hellenistic and Christian thinking with which Hadot concerns himself. As Russell suggests in his history, it is the Christian insistence upon the importance of a 'pure heart', as opposed to any more sophisticated or worldly virtues, which stands it in great contrast to ancient ethics (Russell 1945, p. 111). It is this tension between knowing goodness and simple goodness with which Murdoch wrestles and with which this book is also concerned.

Some have been tempted by the very assessment which Aristotle appears to be warding off, to understand his own ethics as recommending an understanding of ethical life as being highly (even primarily) dependent upon the circumstance, that the 'good life' must also be the 'lucky life'. That, yes, tough as it may seem, the good looking, well-spoken, bodily able, financially wealthy and, most importantly, intellectually capable *man* is indeed the better creature, the one who is better able to lead the 'good life'.[9] Two immediate concerns with this reading of Aristotle's ethics might be raised, first, an exegetical one: that Aristotle, at least, might not, in fact, advocate an evaluation of persons with any significant weight on fortune; and secondly a more fundamental concern: over the accuracy of such a theory regardless of whether or not Aristotle proposed it.[10] It cannot be denied that Aristotle certainly did espouse ethics which placed intellectual activities in pride of place in human existence. Of course, no issue is being taken with any exegesis in this regard, philosophy was (and still is for many) an activity chiefly characterised by contemplation, it is the topmost room of the ivory tower (though it may now frequently invite the natural sciences to share its quarters).[11] The important difference between these ancient and modern perceptions of philosophy which Hadot is pointing out is that whereby the ancient understanding accords the pursuit of 'wisdom' an explicitly ethical character and the modern need not. Modern philosophy (of various kinds) has inherited a means but not an end. The question we must ask is whether philosophy as a 'way of life' is only able to offer an ethical framework which is useful to the academic or whether something more nuanced or complex might be at play. Can εὐδαιμονία be achieved by non-intellectual means?

It seems quite uncontroversial to say that there are people who are not intellectuals in any usual sense, yet who are nevertheless very good people.[12] They might be generous; they might be gentle, brave, kind, loyal, affable, joyful or diligent. There are so many virtues which do not require a quick mind, nor a mind which harbours a great array of knowledge, they require neither the ability nor the inclination to read, nor to investigate abstract problems (perhaps not even to be human). This does not, however, answer any question as to whether someone who has some of these sorts of virtues but is also 'intelligent', is not then better, in some sense, than one who is less intelligent. This certainly seems to be the theory espoused by many ancient philosophers, and one which would seem prevalent still. If one person were brave and another gentle and yet another both brave and gentle, would we not think this third person best? What then if they added some intellectual virtue, would they not then be even better? And mightn't it be fair to suggest that some virtues are more important (morally) than other virtues? If this final condition were permitted, then it may well be uncontroversial (in ancient and modern times) to suggest that intellectual virtue is the most important of all. Intelligence (or something close to what we probably mean by 'intelligence') might be imaged to have further-reaching moral consequences than the other virtues. An understanding of philosophy as a way of life may very well appear to lend itself to just this sort of ethical theory.

Philosophy then becomes a kind of virtue collection activity, with a psychological virtue as its greatest prize.

Even a more typical understanding of philosophy, as an academic activity (in the modern sense of 'academic'), would sit fairly comfortably with this sort of evaluation. Education, commonly conceived, touts academic achievement as a sort of pinnacle of human achievement to which all should aspire and in the light of which people can justly be categorized according to how far they have approached this brilliant peak.[13] In this sense, the asceticism of some ancient schools of philosophy and medieval cloisters is not so distant from many contemporary models of evaluating our achievements. One model offers intelligence as key, the other as simply another excellent (perhaps the best) muscle to flex. To live the life of the mind is the key to being a truly good person.

One might be tempted by the Christian reaction against this intellectualism, as G. K. Chesterton is, and to see the converse as true. By placing the 'pure heart' of which Russell speaks, at the centre of one's ethical evaluation, an emphasis upon the intellect might well be viewed as counterproductive both to this purity and to one's general wellbeing.

> Poetry is sane because it floats easily in an infinite sea; reason seeks to cross the infinite sea, and so make it finite. The result is mental exhaustion...If you argue with a madman, it is extremely probable that you will get the worst of it; for in many ways his mind moves all the quicker for not being delayed by the things that go with good judgement. He is not hampered by a sense of humour or by charity, or by the dumb certainties of experience. He is the more logical for losing certain sane affections. Indeed, the common phrase for insanity is in this respect a misleading one. The madman is not the man who has lost his reason. The madman is the man who has lost everything except his reason.
>
> (Chesterton 1908, p. 16, 19)

Chesteron makes clear that he does not take issue with logic and reason as such, though we do gain the impression that the intellect is, here, viewed as something which should be subservient to a dogma of moral realism and common sense: reason as a handmaiden to revelation. So, by this understanding, adding logical prowess to a list of someone's virtues need not contribute favourably to their ethical worth.

This juxtaposition, between intellectualism and anti-intellectualism, is a crude one. Firstly, imagining that there are only two competing theories of the place of intelligence in our ethical lives supposes that the dichotomy presented is a justified one; between intellect as prince and intellect as a servant. Secondly, this dispute also supposes that the two positions (as sketched above) are dealing with the same subject matter. It is crucial that if any headway is to be made in assessing the role of intelligence in our moral lives, then we must first come to some more sophisticated understanding of what is being referred to by this group of vague cognitive terms: 'intelligence', 'reason', 'logic', 'knowledge', 'rationality', 'mind' and *'wisdom'*. Such terms are thrown around as if it were self-evident what is being referred to. It isn't.

Certainly there is something nebulous which we can recognise, something to do with mental activity as opposed to more tangible pursuits. Many of the aptitudes being highlighted are certainly frequently distinguishable. We often know bright people when we meet them; but are they all of one sort? That seems far less clear. Academia itself appears to be structured around the idea that there are many kinds of intelligence, each with its own niche in which to excel, yet even here there is frequently an attitude of hierarchy.[14]

If philosophy can correctly and fruitfully be understood as a process of self-improvement, and this 'discipline' can and should resemble (at least to some extent) the ancient model which took εὐδαιμονία as its goal, and intellectual excellence as its means, then some suitably robust philosophy of mind and of ethics must be achieved.

To reconcile the sage and the everyman in an evaluative structure which does indeed do justice to them both, it is proposed that a particular study must be made of an idea of 'wisdom', of the way in which there might be an intellectual capacity which is also particularly ethical which encompasses many ideas hitherto highlighted and which can demonstrate both a supremacy amongst virtues and also allow for the equal excellence of the 'pure heart'; an ethic of intellectual virtue which is not just useful to the academic, and which is also an ethic of the 'pure heart' not only of use to the saint or ascetic.

It might be objected that there is some shoehorning going on here, with a desire for a kind of egalitarianism of capacities where there exists no such thing. This charge would, however, suppose that there is no good reason to suggest that there is an intellectual virtue which is of paramount importance to being good whilst also ways of being *just as good* without demonstrating any of the usual virtues associated with intellectual ability. No systematic argument shall be forwarded as to the justice of Murdoch's suggestion. It is hoped that the ethical importance of something which we might call wisdom and of how it stands in relation to other evident virtues and our potential flourishing is conspicuous enough as to, at the very least, permit an investigation. We need only be willing to entertain the idea, at this stage, that there might be some kind of virtue which is 'primus inter pares' amongst other virtues, and that it has something to do with a uniquely broad and penetrating understanding of the world and a tying together of many other virtues. This needn't be something which Socrates achieved perfectly, but rather something towards which he and others like him have pointed. It is enough to ask: 'if there were such a thing as wisdom, what would it be like and how would it work?', then we can better set about seeing how this sort of virtue might fit with our lives and the world in which we live.

Notes

1 Fragment DK119 (22B) of Heraclitus is (as can be expected of any fragment of Heraclytus) very tricky to pin down (Robin Waterfield gives a nice sense of this in his summary of Heraclytus' fragments in (Waterfield 2000, p. 31). Here Waterfield translates 119 as: 'Man's character is his guardian spirit'. Shirley Darcus (Sullivan) offers a good analysis of 'ἔθος' and 'δαιμον' in relation to this fragment in '"Daimon" as a force shaping "Ethos" in Heraclytus' (1974, pp. 390–407). I will translate this fragment as: 'a human's way of life is their spirit'. Most famously, the meaning of this fragment is disputed by Heidegger in his 'Letter on Humanism' (Heidegger 1946, pp. 270–273).

2 Of course, Socrates was not acting in a vacuum. Philosophy as a moral and practical thing was an existing model prior to Socrates. In this way, it may be more accurate to call Socrates a champion rather than a founder or inventor. And it is equally important to recognise that this 'Socratic' model had to contend with the more theoretical and professional model of philosophy even in its ancient forms (John Cooper describes this in *Pursuits of Wisdom* [2013, pp. 27–30]).

3 Larry Siedentop makes the suggestion that Socrates was so much a part of this polis ethic that this is at the root of the conflict with the Sophists, since they did not belong to any particular state in the way that Socrates belonged to Athens and were, therefore, 'amoral' (Siedentop 2014, pp. 43–45).

4 It should also be noted that Nussbaum continues by acknowledging the cumbersome nature of a translation to 'human flourishing' and her own preference for maintaining a transliteration.

5 Kirsten Brukamp, in her tribute to the work of Nussbaum, gives a nice sense of how despite talk of εὐδαιμονία being principally founded in Aristotle's ethics, many Greek authors found common focus in εὐδαιμονία as a purpose of human life even if they did not agree on just what it meant (Brukamp 2000, pp. 93–104).

6 The qualifier 'alternative' is perhaps unnecessary since some therapies which derive (at least in part) from the movement 'back' to the way of life philosophy are quite mainstream. Cognitive Behavioural Therapy is perhaps the most notable and significant element of the 'way of life' movement is concentrated on this explicit relationship between ancient Greek philosophy and modern medicine. Donald Robertson dedicates his volume *The Philosophy of Cognitive Behavioural Therapy* to not only the history of CBT's emergence from ancient Stoicism but also to the wisdom which can still be gleaned from Stoicism in the execution of psychological therapy (Robertson 2010). In part (and to a certain extent), this book resembles more closely the work of Tim LeBon in his effort to withdraw somewhat from the medical impulse of some way of life philosophies (to put philosophy to work in 'healing people'), and to ask whether ethics and learning should have a more central place (LeBon 2001).

7 Hadot is also in pain to emphasise certain differences between the Christian and pagan traditions (*Ibid.*, p. 82).

8 The dates I have given for the authorship of Aristotle's major works are those during which he was resident and teaching in Athens (see Russell 1945, p. 183).

9 Cooper is emphatic about the role of external goods in Aristotle's ethics (Cooper 1985, pp. 173–196). The position here, however, is not to deny that Aristotle discusses the role of external goods in achieving what might be called a well (eudaimon) life, only the importance he gives this in living a life well. Two glasses may both be full whilst one is far bigger than the other; I am only suggesting that Aristotle wants us to be concerned far more with completeness and less with capacity. A very small glass which is well filled is more eudaimon than a big one which is poorly filled.

10   It is the second point which will be of greatest interest here, though the former might be made through attrition rather than concerted effort. Ultimately, it will be suggested that in both cases some confusion has been reached regarding the important distinction between the 'good life' and a 'life lived well'; it is the latter which needs to concern us most in normative ethics, though it is not unrelated to what might also be called the 'desirable life'.

11   On philosophy's place as a chiefly intellectual, contemplative or academic activity associated with the sciences, Thomas Uebel's essay on Neurath's anticipation of naturalised epistemology draws a nice historical line of how this 'handmaiden' philosophy has developed (Uebel 1996, p. 283).

12   It is worth noting a basic sympathy here with the educational psychology and 'multiple intelligences' of the gratifyingly named Howard Gardner (Gardner 1993). So one could talk about moral knowledge as a kind of intelligence (perhaps emotional). I suspect that using the word 'intelligence' in this way can lead to unwelcome confusion and the foundation of this book in ancient ethics means there is no need to use this kind of psychological terminology since talk of 'knowledge' and, more importantly, 'virtues', is far more apt.

13   Self-improvement could be conceived of as the goal of education or learning more generally and the degree to which the metaphilosophy espoused in this book is an effort to reduce (or expand) 'philosophy' to be synonymous with these general concepts constitutes a valid potential addendum. This question will not be explored in explicit depth or detail but the criticism of conventional academic models which is part of this metaphilosophy is certainly commensurate with other commentaries which seek to unravel the academic and competition-orientated 'myth of meritocracy'. As Khen Lampert suggests, the ubiquity with which teachers express a sentiment of unlimited academic potential is often shocking (Lampert 2013, pp. 2–4).

14   James Duderstadt remarks on the ubiquity of this snobbery in relation to the hierarchy of disciplines which is frequently encountered at universities (Duderstadt 2000, p. 123).

Part I
Philosophy

2   Plato and Aristotle on the nature of wisdom

To be honest, as this world goes, is to be one man picked out of ten thousand.

(Shakespeare, *Hamlet*, 2.2)

οὐ καλῶς λέγεις, ὦ ἄνθρωπε, εἰ οἴει δεῖν κίνδυνον ὑπολογίζεσθαι τοῦ ζῆν ἢ τεθνάναι ἄνδρα, ὅυτο τι καὶ σμικρὸν ὄφελμος ἐστιν, ἀλλ᾽ οὐκ ἐκεῖνο μόνον σκοπεῖν, ὅταν πράττῃ, πότερα δίκαια ἢ ἄδικα πράτει, καὶ ἀνδρὸς ἀγαθοῦ ἔργα ἢ κακοῦ.

(Plato, *Apology*, §28, b[1])

εἴπομενδὴ ὅτι οὐκ ἔστιν ἕξις· καὶ γὰρ τῷ καθεύδοντι διὰ βίου ὑπάρχοι ἄν, φυτῶν ζῶντι βίον, καὶ τῷ δυστυχοῦντι τὰ μέγιστα.

(Aristotle, *Nicomachean Ethics*, §X, vi (1176ᵃ, 33–35))[2]

Both Plato and Aristotle agree that the epitome of human life, the most excellent and admirable object to which we might aspire, consists in a psychological virtue. 'σοφία' has, both etymologically and (perhaps to a lesser extent) actively, defined the discipline and life of Western philosophy throughout its history.[3] One might have hoped, then, that a sure port of call in any effort to better understand this concept and its cognates, particularly at its inception, would be these two seminal masters of the subject, these two men who did, between them, establish this debate in earnest. And yet, despite the confidence with which each of these philosophers forwards their wisdom-orientated ethics, and the breadth of the normative claims which are made on the basis of this sophic-primacy, a clear definition of this virtue subsists neither between nor within the principle works of these authors on the subject.

It is undoubtedly important to recognise at the outset that the Nicomachean Ethics and the Apology do, perhaps even more than the other works of Aristotle and Plato which we have, illustrate the different *kinds* of writing which these two men were engaged in. Plato has left us with a corpus of published dialogues, works polished, dramatised and disseminated to a readily consuming audience. Aristotle has not. The Apology is not only a piece of scholarly writing, it is not purely a systematic treatment of what it is to be wise, but it is also a piece of political propaganda, a monument to a mentor, a teacher, a founder and hero. The Nicomachean Ethics[4] is not so varied in style. Aristotle's widely published work has not survived intact and few facts in the history of philosophy are to be so lamented.[5] EN is a far more single-minded treatment of the subject, broad in its remit certainly, almost to the point of being incomparable to Plato's brief depiction of Socrates' trial, but it is an essay on human excellence. Though both works adopt radically differing styles, each serves as a seminal articulation of the nature of wisdom and its status as the ultimate good.

So that we might gain a better understanding, not only of the history of theories of wisdom, but also of the concept as it stands and its importance in contemporary ethics, it is certainly important to explore what both of these texts say on the subject and, if possible, how they might complement one another. Needless to say, it is not necessary to attempt an exposition of Aristotle's entire theory of the ultimate good but it is important to recognise that it is a complex theory which involves a range of concepts which are inextricably linked and mutually defined, in fact, this is simultaneously a significant strength of Aristotle' theory of wisdom and a major weakness.

The brutal simplicity of Plato's ethical specifications, exemplified by his suggestion that a good person cannot be concerned with danger to his life, strikes us as intuitively wrong. It could only be an ethic suitable for ascetics, saints and martyrs (and only then, very judgmental ones). At the same time, Aristotle's suggestion that fortune is vital to the ethical worth of a human being can seem overly harsh and, perhaps more importantly, instructively vacuous. Yet, Plato's insistence on basic ethical reflection as being at the core of wisdom and the good life may seem to point in a positive direction and the importance which Aristotle gives to practical concerns and the manifold vagaries of life similarly so. It is in these areas, then, that this discussion seeks some degree of resolution and clarity, in the suggestion that whilst the Apology and EN are mutually critical in some respects, they are also beneficial to one another through that criticism and in agreement in other important respects.

Investigating any theory of wisdom (and, for that matter, any other expansive concept) must contend with the difficulty of appropriately disentangling and conflating related concepts. To fully justify any approach to doing this would require a separate and extensive discussion; what is important to do here is make clear that although various psychological virtues, states and activities are discussed by both Plato and Aristotle, the latter author does far more to distinguish, and the former far more to conflate. The current discussion follows Emmanuel Ackah in appraising the Socratic theory of virtue as a whole, not only with moral knowledge and wisdom being synonymous (a more widely accepted conflation) but also, and more importantly, with wellbeing also forming a central part of this ethico-epistemological state (Ackah 2003, p. 124). Ackah contrasts his own theory with not only

an established understanding of Socrates' principal activity as being normative but also with that of Hugh Benson, who insists that Socrates also
engages in an epistemological exercise (*Ibid.*, p. 123).[6] Benson does not deny,
of course, that Socrates is mainly concerned with ethics, only that he is also
and distinctly concerned with how we appreciate the truth. It is this distinction which Ackah criticises and which is most important here. Are knowing
and being unrelated for Plato? Can a wise person be a bad person? Perhaps
Alexander Nehamas is correct in identifying some fault in the tradition,
which Benson follows, of refusing to expand any interpretation of Plato's
theory any distance beyond Socrates' words (Nehamas 2001, p. 719). We
may well need to read between the lines and appreciate Plato as an author
of philosophy more than Socrates as a historical philosopher, in order to
propose an interpretation of Plato as espousing a cohesive theory of ethical
and epistemological holism. That's what Ackah does, that's what this discussion does.

The Apology

So, the rumour had got about that Socrates thought himself the wisest man
of them all. No doubt this sort of claim, when made about someone who
repeatedly and openly criticised people of high social standing, would inevitably cause many individuals a good deal of agitation. It would certainly
put these highfalutin folks in a mood to push this trouble maker into a tight
spot, enough that he would be forced to make a public denunciation of this
rumour. No such luck. Instead Plato shows us an unrepentant, casual, clever
old man who explains the Delphic origins of this rumour and the probable
meaning of the divine proclamation.

Socrates is wisest because he is the only person who seems to know that
he doesn't know anything at all (*Apol.*, §21ᵈ). Certainly, Plato is aware of the
contradiction being stated here, and it falls together nicely with the irreverent yet open and honest humour Socrates possesses throughout the proceedings. It is not that Socrates doesn't mean what he is saying, but he does
mean more than he is saying. It is not that he doesn't know anything *as
such*, only that he doesn't know anything which should elevate him above
others; his knowledge is not something divine, *it is not complete knowledge,
but rather it is the wisdom of a lived human life.* Far from a boast, Socrates
begins to sound self-deprecating. "Human wisdom is of little or no value";
this is what the oracle's words must have meant, Socrates tells us, and that
he is simply an example of someone who recognises this truth (*Ibid.*, 23ᵃ).
Socrates has already told us that he may indeed be wise but that this wisdom is of a different character from the sort of thing he is being accused
of, he does not claim some kind of intimate knowledge of the nature of the
cosmos, some complete and comprehensive certainty regarding an ultimate
reality (which undoubtedly does exist but which is not for human minds to
comprehend) instead he has something else, he has 'ἀνθρωπίνη σοφία'.

Surely though, we cannot accept that Socrates is being honest if on the one hand, he is claiming that this human wisdom is worthless and at other times is exercising aspects of this wisdom through ethical instruction which he clearly believes to be of the greatest importance. Socrates, in fact, knows what is 'the greatest good for humans', 'μέγιστον ἀγαθὸν ὂν ἀνθρώπῳ', he knows it to be *criticism* (*Ibid.*, 38ª).[7] As Sharon Ryan points out, some have considered Socrates' humility to be itself definitive of wisdom (Ryan, 1999, p. 119), yet how are we to take this 'humility' seriously when it is followed by such wanton judgement and instruction? In what sense is Socrates humble?

Again, it can be salutary to remind oneself that what is being read is itself a philosophical text, one in which Socrates voices not only his own (possible) words but also (and primarily) those of his pupil. It seems doubtful that Plato was either malicious or stupid enough to portray his mentor and friend as a contradictory oaf, rather, it would seem fairer to suggest that Socrates is pointing towards different kinds of importance, different scales of understanding and truth. The charge of wisdom which Socrates denies is evidently being contrasted with the kind of ethical, 'human wisdom' which Socrates is claiming. Socrates suggests that Apollo probably does possess the kind of wisdom which he does not and this may well lead us to believe that this superior form of wisdom is something fanciful, a red herring allowing for Socrates to then construct a false modesty around an intelligible form of wisdom (*Apol.*, 23ª).

Yet, allowing for Plato's integrity and intelligence in this matter, we might rather suppose that this superior wisdom is simply a broader form of intellectual achievement, a kind of general scientific knowledge and certain, metaphysical insight of the sort pursued by many Pre-Socratic thinkers (Roochnik 2004, p. 19, 64). Socrates does not know what the first principle of the universe is, nor does he profess to know the nature of the gods, in fact, he very frequently doesn't know the answer to the ethical and psychological questions in which he engages. All he knows is that *it is vital to ask these questions*, that it is important to be a good person and that there are some particular virtues which it is important to possess in order to be a good person (amongst which are inquisitiveness and open-mindedness).

Very general principles of human life, that is what Socrates can recognise. Of course, some modern philosophers might restrict the remit of their discipline even further, with an understanding that metaphysics is essentially meaningless, but Socrates does not do this. It's not that Socrates doesn't believe in the objects of cosmic wisdom, he categorically does (for he denies the charges of atheism being levelled against him), nor does he suggest that such wisdom is impossible (or utterly detached from human wisdom), he simply doubts the possibility for humans to possess such perfect wisdom, at least as a cohesive whole. Instead, we must pursue most urgently those glimpses of truth that are available to us.

It is not, then, that human wisdom is different in epistemological *type* from other wisdom, it is still the comprehension of truth, objective and real, it is just far less exhaustive than an understanding of the nature of the cosmos and all that is in it, it is a small part of a grand whole. So, in comparison to the kind of wisdom which philosophers had sought prior to Socrates, the sort which Socrates was being accused of, his own understanding of his own limitations and a few broad ethical truths is, in an important sense, very little. Even compared to the level of knowledge professed by non-philosophers, those who practice crafts (particularly statecraft) for instance, with their libraries of certainties and pedagogical bravado, the understanding that such confidence is flawed is still humbler than if such confidence were not flawed.

Undoubtedly this claim is made by Socrates with some degree of tongue-in-cheek provocation. In relation to the wisdom of a god, Socrates' wisdom is insignificant. In the grand scheme of things, objectively speaking, this human wisdom is only a wee scrap of a thing. Indeed, *if* all these distinguished gentlemen who see fit to accuse Socrates of corrupting the youth of Athens were in fact in possession of the wisdom which they profess then, similarly, Socrates' ethical and epistemological insights would be relatively limited. But it is big *if*. They are not in possession of this greater wisdom and Socrates knows this. His denial is not without its humorous barb, nor should it be, for, in making his defense, Socrates also wishes to demonstrate the principal aspect of this human wisdom.

As aforementioned, Socrates indicates that the core of his wisdom lies in criticism, in the 'examined life', in a relentless pursuit of truth, honesty and the good life (*Apol.*, 38ᵃ). Nor is this duty a solitary one, and this is what has got Socrates into trouble, he wishes to engage others in this activity:

> And if any of you argues the point, and says he does care, I shall question and examine and cross-examine him, and if I find that he does not possess virtue, but says he does, I shall rebuke him for scorning the things that are of most importance and caring more for what is of less worth. This I shall do to whomever I meet, young and old, foreigner and citizen...
>
> (*Ibid.*, 29ᵉ–30ᵃ)

Quite strong stuff. There might even be part of a modern reader who begins to sympathise with Socrates' accusers. It is all well and good making the whimsical analogy of a horsefly but the previous analogy which Socrates makes of the warrior might be nearer the mark (*Ibid.*, 30ᵉ; 28ᵃ–29ᵇ). Persistence is one thing, but aggression and bloody-minded devotion are quite another.

Must we ask ourselves, then, whether Socrates invokes Achilles as a paragon of philosophic virtue for the benefit of his accusers or whether Plato does so to describe a theory of wisdom? Or perhaps the point is somewhat more complex. It is the courage in the face of death which these warriors demonstrate which Socrates praises, and we must surely recognise that not only would the real Socrates have been well aware of his intentions at his trial and the imminent threat of death with which he was presented, but Plato too would want us to be aware of the soldierly bravery which his mentor exhibited throughout his life. These men of Athens executed not only the wisest man in Greece but also a brave Athenian soldier. What fools! Yet both Socrates and Plato evidently believed that this virtue of courage played an important role in either achieving or forming wisdom itself.

If wisdom is viewing and enacting accurately those few, small, ethical truths which we might appreciate, then it may well follow that there are certain struggles involved in reaching this goal and that other virtues are required to overcome them. So when Socrates professes that 'it is not hard to escape death; it is much harder to escape wickedness, for that runs faster than death' (*Ibid.*, 39ᵃ), the courage for which he calls is not only in the face of death, it is the courage required beyond that, the courage to fight the battles on one's own less bloody battlefields. And if the metaphor of war is an uncomfortable one for a modern reader then we must not only be wary of anathema, but also of disregarding an important arena of human activity; of vices, yes, but also virtues. These men of Athens needn't have dealt with death as an abstract pawn of thought experiments, creeping in the shadows of retirement homes and half-forgotten funerals, they had war ready to hand.

So here (Socrates says) is an obvious kind of courage, but don't ignore some other more important kinds. And of course he is right. When you stand there in the thick of conversation with those both known and unknown and suddenly a travesty of foolishness and misinformation spews forth from an unfortunate mouth; they have made a simple error of information perhaps, or even worse they have made an immoral conviction clear. Who hasn't experienced the sudden call for courage, the pressing need to judge a complex battlefield of social expectations for weaknesses and opportunities? And countless other daily skirmishes of the soul, less public, which call for bravery without glory? To halt one's hand or to press it into action. To break that conversation with an uncomfortable question. And who has not faltered? Of course, Plato is right. But it is still a bit much.

This is not Troy and the gods do not fight restlessly by our sides. We are not Achilles nor should we expect to be. Despite the need, perhaps quite urgent need in some cases, to instill in ourselves and others greater honesty, critical reflection and moral courage, it need not follow that someone who experiences fear of death has no ethical worth whatsoever. This just feels like throwing the baby out with the bathwater.

We are reminded again of Murdoch claiming that 'an unexamined life can be virtuous' (Murdoch 1970, pp. 1–2). Not only are there manifold ways of demonstrating virtue, but there are also at least as many situations which one might encounter which alter the ethical battlefield dramatically. A gentle, loving, kind and generous person may yet cower when you point a gun at them. Even more importantly, this virtuous person might fluctuate in their inclinations. *Mood is master of much*; and whilst they may frequently be generous they may not be diligent, temperate, let alone bright and certainly not incessantly so. Supposing that Susan Wolf is correct in suggesting that we should neither expect nor desire moral sainthood in ourselves or those we care about (Wolf 1982, pp. 419–439), does Plato's theory of wisdom, as presented in the Apology, offer any defense against such charges of extremism? Well, perhaps it is a matter of orientation and perspective.

Socrates professes that his keenest desire is to help people to become better (*Apol.*, 24–26). He has identified the way we can be better human beings and that is to be critical and reflexive and to foster ethical virtues in ourselves. He wishes to show his fellow Athenians the truth of this by breaking down their assumptions and narrow view of the world; to see their own small place in the great scheme of things and their own limited responsibilities. He wishes for them to focus on what is really important to them: their ethical selves. 'Virtue does not come from money, but from virtue comes money and all other good things to man' (*Ibid.*, 30ᵇ). So, whilst we may not be inclined to accept Socrates' theory, of how to be the best one can be, in its strongest form, we may yet recognise the importance of the direction it urges us to face. The Athenians whom Socrates addresses and to whom Plato wrote were in danger of having their attention stolen by a narrow world of the profession and social climbing, of wealth and personal physical wellbeing; Socrates wishes to turn their minds to a wider vision of the world and their own true places in it. We are ethical beings first and foremost and all other concerns must be cast in this light. For Socrates, it is this honest perspective on things and action based upon it which constitutes both the essence of human wisdom and the means for good living in general. We might, then, allow for this kind of wisdom to be a not particularly intellectual form of virtue. Of course, it is presented to us in this way, but it would seem fair to suggest that a certain kind of broad perspective and consequent humility, coupled with an ethical orientation could be at the core of all virtuous persons and that this sort of wisdom is far from elitist.

Nicomachean Ethics

But are our lives so simple that we can simply turn away from daily concerns? Is ethical conduct so straightforward as to require a single orientation? Aristotle's Nicomachean Ethics sets forth an alternative perspective whereby the intellectual virtues are divided into sufficient categories that another form of wisdom is allowed for. Φρόνησις is a tandem virtue to σοφία, one which involves a practical awareness of the complex variety of situations in which virtues (and vices) can be exercised and the clarity of thought and judgement to pursue the best course (*EN*, §VI, v; 1140ᵃ24–1140ᵇ30). It is perhaps to be expected that Aristotle departs from Plato in moving away from a theory whereby abstract and occasionally intangible universals serve as a source of inspiration and towards a system that takes real-life scenarios as the sources of virtue and vice.[8] Aristotle says comparatively little about σοφία in the *EN* and we might be fooled into thinking that this more traditional conception of wisdom is unimportant and that φρόνησις has taken its place. It may be worthwhile, however, keeping in mind that φρόνησις is not simply a discreet capacity isolated from other intellectual virtues.

Φρόνησις is indeed one of five such virtues listed by Aristotle: 'τέχνη, ἐπιστήμη, φρόνησις, σοφία, νοῦς' (*EN*, §VI, v; 1140ᵃ24–1140ᵇ30). It may be worth keeping these terms in Greek (or transliterated), as tomes could be written merely attempting to translate these words into English. They might be translated roughly as: 'technical skill' (or knowing how to make by sound judgement), 'scientific skill' (or knowing a fact by sound deductive reasoning and observation), 'prudence' (knowing what's best by sound deliberation on one's own wellbeing), 'wisdom' (knowing a fundamental fact by sound deductive and inductive reasoning; though this may combine *all* virtues, not just science and intelligence) and 'intelligence' (knowing a fact by sound inductive reasoning). These virtues do not, by any means, exhaust the psychological capabilities and qualities of human beings, they are, rather, the means by which one comes to understand truth.[9]

It is immediately apparent that Aristotle's treatment of wisdom differs dramatically from Plato's. Both authors were dealing with a Greek world struggling to understand their occupation, though each treats this task in a very different way. Where Plato's Socrates rejects the vast majority of intellectual baggage and pretense which 'wisdom' carries with it, Aristotle seeks to pick up the pieces and sort them into some kind of sensible order. Neither departs from the general idea that they are systematic truth-seekers, one simply suggests that the only appropriate truth-seeking to be done is in the destruction of false preconceptions and the pursuit of right and moral action; the other that a wide variety of truth can be pursued and that moral action is dependent upon individual circumstances and an ability to judge those circumstances (or so it seems at first glance).

This summary might give the impression that there is very little room for reconciling the two views, even in part, and yet, as aforementioned, Aristotle's theory is complex and extensive. It is clear at least, and Aristotle says so explicitly, that the virtue which he calls σοφία is actually a combination of two of the other virtues: scientific skill and intelligence (*EN*, §VI, vii; 1141a:19–21). This sort of wisdom is the most general and holistic, it is all knowledge tied together in its most complete and perfect form, it is true authority, it is exactly the sort of thing Socrates was denying possession of. Aristotle is adamant that σοφία is necessarily general and, as such, must be distinguished from the kind of ethical insight which characterises good people which must, due to the sheer variety of characters, lives and species, be more adaptable and personalised.

> It is also clear that wisdom cannot be the same thing as knowledge about people; for if we are to call knowledge about our own interests wisdom, there will be a number of different kinds of wisdom, one for

each species: there cannot be a single such wisdom dealing with the good of all living things, any more than there is one art of medicine for all existing things.

(*EN*, §VI, vii; 1141a:29–33)[10]

For this reason, Aristotle explains, there must be another form of wisdom, one which concerns how to be a good human and this he calls φρόνησις. It is tempting, and quite possibly accurate to assume at this stage that Aristotle is simply fleshing out Plato's theory of wisdom and giving a name to the Socratic 'human wisdom' to better distinguish it from σοφία. We might be inclined to think that the two theories are, in fact, very similar indeed, yet there remains an apparent gulf between these authors' attitudes towards the nature of goodness itself.

Aristotle's ethical relativism has been interpreted in various ways. Some commentators have read passages like that quoted above to support a cultural relativist view.[11] Commandeering virtue ethics and Aristotle for the cause of cultural relativism may, however, say more about a zeitgeist than it does Aristotle, and it certainly seems less of a stretch to limit Aristotle to biological relativism. This is the approach of Martha Nussbaum and it would appear, ostensibly at least, to be a fair one (Nussbaum 1998, pp. 271–274).

Aristotle discusses the customs of Greeks of previous times, calling them 'simple and barbaric' and claims that 'In general, all men seek not the way of their forefathers, but rather, the good' (*Politics* §II, viii; 1269ᵃ:3–4). Of course, exegesis aside, one might argue against both the cultural relativist and the biological relativist on the basis of their following Aristotle's tradition of making use of arbitrary and sweeping generalisations (regarding either 'cultures' or 'species').[12] It would seem quite legitimate to question how far Aristotle's own idea of humanity stretched. Slaves? Women? Barbarians? Other primates?[13] It would seem wise, in fact, to keep Aristotle's own dictum of precision appropriate to subject matter in our minds when considering the vastness and complexity of both human cultures and other living things (*EN*, §I, iii; 1194ᵇ:13–27). We might, however (whilst keeping a weather eye on family resemblance) allow for some nebulous categories (of whatever nature) to be valid sources of inspiration for ethical considerations.[14]

Such an allowance would certainly strengthen the case against the commensurability of Plato and Aristotle's theories of wisdom. There is something which we call human and it seems entirely reasonable to suggest there is a roughly definable collection of ways in which this human being can flourish. This may indeed vary here and there but there is certainly a core collection of virtues that can be identified. Indeed, Aristotle's φρόνησις allows for just this sort of variation as this practical sense allows for someone to judge just what is appropriate for themselves as a distinct member of their species and community who encounters novel situations. It is primarily this necessity for a form of ethical wisdom which takes account of the (often seemingly trivial) minutiae of an individual life which drives both

Aristotle and Plato to distance this form of wisdom from an understanding of general principles of the cosmos. And yet both authors refuse to sever ethical thinking from general principles.

It is at this point of Aristotle's consideration of how to be a good human being that he becomes most confusing. Again this is almost certainly due in part to the unpolished nature of the text (at §VI, ix, it becomes particularly fractured). Critically, however, Aristotle focuses on the kind of thinking which sound ethical deliberation consists of and he acknowledges that an evil human could be crafty and accurate in considerations of their own well-being to some extent and yet we would be wrong to call this person wise in any sense. Aristotle thus concludes that φρόνησις consists in a species of the soundness of mind, a kind of habit of thought, attitude, awareness and action *which leads to goodness* (*EN*, §VI, xii; 1144a:36–7).

This is not a strictly cognitive process with a conclusion which can be called true or false, but rather 'being correct in the sense of arriving at something good'. So whilst φρόνησις need not be directly concerned with general principles it must nevertheless conform to non-instrumental ideas of goodness to some extent. In fact, Aristotle also explains the further intellectual virtue of 'understanding', which is the sound judgement required to perceive the right opinions which can lead to sound deliberation (*EN*, §VI, x; 1142b:36-1143a:19). Indeed it becomes apparent that all of these virtues are tied together and Aristotle gradually becomes more and more inclusive in his consideration of these virtues. Despite the insistence upon distinction, even σοφία and φρόνησις are intimately linked to the extent that φρόνησις *leads to* σοφία (*EN*, §VI, xiii; 1145a:7-11). Indeed, σοφία is revealed to be something far more than simply comprehending some abstract, metaphysical insights, it is the fulcrum about which all virtue and human wellbeing pivot, it is certainly a far more pervasive thing than first suggested (*EN*, §VI, vii; 1141a:9-1141b:23). Aristotle is perhaps most perspicuous when he engages his medical analogies for it is in this way that he explains that:

> ...it is not really the case that φρόνησις is in authority, over Σοφία or over the higher part of the intellect, any more than medical science is in authority over health. Medical science does not control health, but studies how to procure it; hence it issues orders in the interests of health, not *to* health.
>
> (*EN*, §VI, xiii; 1145a:7-11)

Φρόνησις is the sensitive and calculative part of our minds. It is the judgemental eye cast over the world. But *this eye could simply be crafty and manipulative; this sight must be guided by good virtue to be a force worth calling any kind of wisdom* (*Ibid.*). It must be searching for and engaging in the right thing. And since σοφία appears to be an activity of being excellent (in the most general and pervasive, if overridingly cognitive, sense) one must have something of this σοφία to be virtuous and therefore to have φρόνησις.

Φρόνησις looks for ways to be good, σοφία is (in part) the activity of being good, but one must already be partly good in order to correctly look for goodness. 'σοφία is part of virtue as a whole, and therefore by its possession, or rather by its exercise, renders a person well' (*EN*, §VI, xii; 1144ᵃ:4-6).

Perhaps the most pressing concern that might be raised concerning this furious mix of psychological phenomena is the manner in which divisions and connections, dependencies and interdependencies are articulated so briefly and forcefully that insufficient clarification is given regarding the nature of this admixture. Why is it so important that Socrates was wrong (so Aristotle tells us) about virtues being principles as opposed to operating in conjunction with principles? This suggestion is certainly heavily predicated upon Aristotle's own strict theory of human psychology and the division of the soul into distinct aspects: higher and lower, intellectual and biological (*De Anima*, §III, viii; 431ᵇ:20-432ᵃ:13).

Yet, mightn't we allow for a more nuanced psychology, one which allows for far greater fluidity and lack of categorical definition? Aristotle certainly indicates this in pointing to the unity of virtues and it is perhaps here that we may find a final possibility for a kernel of an ancient theory of wisdom which accounts for ethical focus and insight, real-life adaptability, holistic understanding and soundness of mind and attitude.

Elizabeth Telfer finds that Aristotle's theory of the unity of virtue requires a 'well-disposedness' and that whilst this is not explicitly claimed as part of Aristotle's theory, it is nevertheless required by it (Telfer 1989–1990, p. 43). Perhaps we could be more generous to Aristotle than Telfer and find that he does indeed suggest this, particularly when he claims that:

> A man of deficient self-restraint or a bad man may as a result of calculation arrive at the object he proposes as the right thing to do, so that he will have deliberated correctly, although he will have gained something extremely evil.
>
> (*EN*, §VI, ix; 1142ᵇ:18-20)

So φρόνησις must be guided by the right sort of desire: by virtue. It cannot be called wisdom unless it is driven by a general kind of goodness, otherwise, as aforementioned, it is just cleverness. Yet Telfer also finds that Aristotle fails to argue successfully for the unity of virtue due to the lack of nuance given to the virtues which must be united, someone may well possess this 'well-disposedness' but they're clearly not going to be perfectly virtuous in every way just because they have φρόνησις (Telfer 1989–1990, p. 46).

Telfer is certainly correct that Aristotle very often presents a vision of a moral world in which virtues can either be possessed perfectly or not at all, but this may be more to do with tone, or mode of expression, than the content of the theory. Certainly, Aristotle's insistence upon time and experience being key to forming φρόνησις (and σοφία) would suggest otherwise (*EN*, §VI,xi; 1143ᵃ:19-1143ᵇ:17). Aristotle certainly isn't suggesting that there is a critical point of age or experience which suddenly grants wisdom, it is, rather, a process of gaining a broader perspective which, in turn, grants both a better appreciation of the means of achieving goodness and fuller participation in and understanding of that goodness itself. So if we can allow for this gradual development of virtues, including φρόνησις and σοφία, then it seems entirely reasonable to suggest that if someone is to be 'called good without qualification' (*EN*, §VI, xiii; 1145ᵃ:1), that is, *not 'good without fault' but simply a 'good person'*, they must possess a cohesive awareness of both the general goodness towards which they strive and an awareness of the relationships between not only their actions and the world around them but also between one virtue and another.

We can imagine someone who is very protective of their family, perhaps even generous with them, yet due to their lack of cohesive moral character and perception of the moral world in which they live, they might also be quite violent or deceitful. This might represent an example of isolated virtue, but it is not *true virtue*. True virtue comes from a virtuous whole and when accompanied by experience and an ever-improving ethical awareness and participation will impact virtue as a whole. It is important to keep in mind that Aristotle speaks of φρόνησις and σοφία as activities, or rather qualities which can be exercised, as opposed to static states. *Φρόνησις is the ability to recognise and participate in good things. Σοφία is the ability to recognise and participate in (amongst other things) virtue(s).* So if we are to believe Aristotle, σοφία is a necessary but not sufficient condition of φρόνησις and φρόνησις is a sufficient but not necessary condition of σοφία. So we can have absent-minded geniuses who we might call wise but who do not understand or participate in particulars.

Aristotle wrestles with a clear need to describe a system of moral virtue and psychological activity which is at once contiguous and cohesive and at the same time composed of distinct aspects. He disagrees with the Socratic vision of moral and intellectual activity which is homogenous and unitary because of its failure to deal with clear differences observed in the world. The wisdom gained through experience and time; the distinctions between those who are naturally good-hearted and those who have a more complete understanding of their ethical activities; the myriad ways in which people can fail or succeed in acting virtuously. Yet he sees the need to describe a system which can also account for the interconnectedness, even singularity, of ethical character and the importance (albeit at a very basic level) of general principals of good and evil, of right and wrong, to act as a foundation of ethical action.

This is where Aristotle's theory of wisdom diverges most completely from Plato's. Socratic 'human wisdom' is not different in *kind* from other wisdom but in *degree*. Socrates is still the wisest man because, not only does he recognise the limits of his own knowledge but also, his recognition of and participation in those more worldly matters which it is our prerogative to understand is more complete. These ethical things occupy a narrower end of the wisdom scale but they lie nevertheless on the same scale. Aristotle demands a more complete division, ethical concerns are particular, active and petty, perhaps they co-operate with grander, more static principals but they exercise a completely different part of our minds.

Plato too argues for the unity of virtue. It is in the *Protagoras* that the Socratic unity of virtue is most fully articulated (*Protagoras*, §329ᶜ6) and as Brickhouse and Smith explain, this theory has divided scholars persistently (Brickhouse and Smith 1997, p. 312). Do Plato's dialogues endorse a view of Virtue as a singular thing expressed in different ways in different circumstances or as a multifaceted thing composed of distinct virtues which can and do form parts of both virtues as a whole and of one another?

This discussion follows Brickhouse and Smith (1997, pp. 312–313) in the suggestion that Plato's account is not as fragmentary or troublesome as this part/whole debate would suggest but rather that Virtue is singular due to the overarching nature of one enveloping virtue, namely σοφία. Different virtues are united through their relation to σοφία, it is through knowledge of good and evil as such that all other virtues exist and are exercised. Aristotle may have deemed that the relationship between this knowledge and it is being exercised (and not being exercised) in particular circumstances was not fully developed by Plato, leaving this abstract master virtue floating in an offputtingly intangible æther. A fair criticism. Yet both authors discuss σοφία not only as an abstract, rarified knowledge of the ultimate principals of the cosmos but also as a kind of lynchpin to good activity.

Both Aristotle and Plato find themselves drawn away from this ethical dimension of σοφία. Aristotle uses a distinct psychological activity as a kind of buffer zone, a cunning slave to spare σοφία the degradation of being associated with the lowly matters of daily human existence; Plato merely sidesteps the need for this association and places himself at the inconsequential fringes of σοφία, a distant admirer, staring longingly at the brilliant core of this cosmic light. For both Plato and Aristotle, true σοφία is not only the preserve of the gods but it is also highly conceptual in nature. Σοφία may be expansive and it may include ethical activity, a life lived 'well-spirited' or 'happily' (either distantly or indirectly) but it is ultimately an intellectual thing.

Not only does Aristotle tell us that 'a life of virtuous activity will essentially be one of eudaimonia' but also that 'eudaimonia is some form of contemplation' (*EN*, §X, viii; 1178ᵇ:20-4). Indeed, since it is this thinking man, this man who 'pursues intellectual activity' who comes closest to divinity, who is most like the gods themselves, this is yet 'another proof that the wise man is most eudaimon'[15]

Plato's ideal may be more religious and less scientific, but he too points to excellence which finds its epitome less in the realm of action and more in the realm of pondering. Given their grand efforts to describe the less abstract sides of psychological virtue both Plato and Aristotle cannot help but ascribe the shining essence of this all-encompassing master virtue to something distinctly rarefied.

It may well be, however, that this contemplative focus of σοφία is less integral to these theories of wisdom than their authors suggest. Indeed, it is this high esteem for intellectualism and its strict division from more worldly concerns which is at the heart of both Aristotle's complex and problematic categorisation and Plato's esoteric intangibility. If we were to allow for a downgrading of this aspect of wisdom, and more complex and messy psychology which does not demand a capacity to deal with such things in isolation, we may well be able to reconcile these theories, not only with one another but also with an acceptable and enlightening view of wisdom more generally. Such a holistic and equitable view may well demand that the relationship between human wisdom, or φρόνησις, and σοφία is biconditional (in line with Plato rather than Aristotle) and it may also demand a potentially uncomfortable tethering of metaphysics and ethics, incompatible with many modern trends of thought, but it would allow for a theory which encompasses ethical focus and insight, real-life adaptability, holistic understanding and soundness of mind and attitude. If there is a kernel to an Aristotelian and Platonic theory of wisdom which can offer insight, it may be found only through this non-intellectual modification. Indeed Aristotle likewise finishes his discussion of wisdom and wellbeing with a hint in this direction, with a tempering of theory through experience:

> ... but it is by the practical experience of life and conduct that the truth is really tested, since it is there that the final decision lies. We must therefore examine the conclusions we have advanced by bringing them to the test of the facts of life. If they are in harmony with the facts, we may accept them... Perhaps however, as we maintain, in the practical sciences the end is not to attain a theoretic knowledge of the various subjects but rather to carry out our theories in action. If so, to know what virtue is is not enough; we must endeavour to possess and to practice it...
>
> (*EN*, §X, viii; 1179ª:20-2, 1179ª:35-1179ᵇ:2)

Perhaps, then, we might ask whether the lived experience of striving to live well reflects the erudite penchants of Aristotle and Plato or whether, as Aristotle was seemingly prepared to accept, wisdom might be spoken of as more inclusive appreciation of goodness in a much broader and less academically centred range of practices.

Notes

1 'You do not speak well, Sir, if you hold that a man ought to be concerned with the danger of life or death, if he is to be of any small worth, rather than that he should look to this alone: when he does things, whether they are right or wrong, and whether they are the actions of a good man or bad.' Though the translation is original it has made particular use of H. N. Fowler's (1966) translation. This instance takes a more literal line and attempts to convey something of Socrates' slightly irreverent tone.

2 'We have said, then, that it [wellbeing] is not a state of being, for if it were it might belong to one who slept though their whole life, or who lived as a vegetable, or someone who suffered great misfortunes'. As above the translation is original though, in this case makes use of Rackham's (1934). For the Nicomachean Ethics, referencing follows the Thomist tradition of book and chapter in addition to Bekker numbers; Plato will use only Stephanus pagination. Other works by Aristotle are given by formats appropriate to the edition used, though often in this dual format.

3 Pierre Hadot (1995, pp. 16–21) discusses the centrality of the idea of Sophia in his discussion of the origins of the activity of philosophy in *What is Ancient Philosophy*. This discussion also follows Hadot in the suggestion that the sometimes imagined dichotomy between sophia as knowledge and sophia as concerned with ethics and wellbeing is, in fact, a false dichotomy.

4 Henceforth 'EN'.

5 On these different kinds of writing and the loss of Aristotle's published works and Plato's lecture notes, see (Copleston 1947, pp. 133–41, 268–276). Copleston highlights here the historical importance of what we have retained and what we have lost from these two great authors.

6 Undoubtedly Ackah's work owes some significant debt to Benson's, not only for a title but also for Benson's critical efforts in bringing Plato's epistemology to the fore (Benson 2000, p. 4).

7 Or 'Examination'.

8 On Aristotle's movement away from Plato's thinking, see Case's (1925, pp. 80–86) *The Development of Aristotle*.

9 Aristotle also expands upon his theory of understanding truth and the importance of observed demonstrations in the *Posterior Analytics* though there he concentrates far more on the role of observation in knowledge (pp. 114–166).

10 This is again based upon Rackham's translation although his translation of πολιτικὴ as 'political science' (here 'knowledge about people') veers somewhat from the tone of this piece and the manner in which Aristotle uses the term very closely with φρόνησις. Aristotle does later develop this relationship, at which point it becomes far clearer what this distinctively political virtue is concerned with (*EN*, §VI, viii; 1141b:23–1142a30).

11 Alisdair MacIntyre does, it must be said, recognise the biological grounds for Aristotle's claims though maintains that it is fair to dismiss these and retain his ethics of virtue for cultural relativism (MacIntyre 1998, p. 287). See also Martha Nussbaum's comments on this (Nussbaum 1998, p. 260).

12 On the arbitrary nature of both species and cultural boundaries, see Samantha Hurn's (2012, pp. 202–219) *Humans and Other Animals*.

13 Of course, Aristotle's grasp of the life sciences was extraordinary but both it and our own must be viewed (appropriately enough) in the light of significant cultural influences. Franz deWaal (2001, p. 359) gives a good sense of the impact of cultural influences on the life sciences in *The Ape and the Sushi Master*.

14 When concerned with definition and distinction it is always wise to keep in mind Wittgenstein's thoughts on the similarities between nebulous entities (Wittgenstein 1953, §67).

15 ὥστε κἂν οὕτως εἴη ὁ σοφὸς μάλιτ᾽ εὐδαίμων (*EN*, §X, viii; 1179a:30–31).

3 Moderate realism as the epistemic and metaethical basis of wisdom

There is Nothing Either Good or Bad, but Thinking Makes it So.
(Shakespeare, *Hamlet*, 2.2)

There are some who, as we have said, both themselves assert that it is possible for the same thing to be and not to be, and say that people can judge this to be the case... Further, it follows that all would then be right and all would be in error, and our opponent himself confesses himself to be in error. And at the same time our discussion with him is evidently about nothing at all; for he says nothing. For he says neither 'yes' nor 'no'; and again he denies both of these and says 'neither yes nor no'; for otherwise there would already be something definite.
(Aristotle, *Metaphysics*, IV, 1005b31–1006a2, 1008a29–34)

Let us assume with Protagoras that your judgement is true for *you*. But isn't it possible that the rest of us may criticize (sic) your verdict?... Secondly, it has this most exquisite feature: Protagoras admits, I presume, that the contrary opinion about his own opinion (namely that it is false) must be true, seeing that he agrees that all men judge what is.
(Plato, *Theatetus*, 170d–171b)

The victorious one, through knowledge Of reality and unreality, In the Discourse to Katyayana, Refuted both 'it is' and 'it is not'.
...
Action depends upon the agent. The agent itself depends on action. One cannot see any way To establish them differently.
(Nagarjuna, *Mulamadhyamakakarika*, XV, 7 and VIII, 12)

Quite a muddle. Someone must be wrong here. But then again, if philosophers like Siddhārtha Gautama and (latterly) Nagarjuna are correct, then perhaps they can all be right and all be wrong at once. But that's not really what these Buddhist philosophers are saying, is it? Perhaps saying 'neither yes nor no' is importantly different from saying nothing at all.

The idea of wisdom highlighted thus far, of a virtue which ties together all virtues, which is cognitive yet not necessarily intellectual, and crucially one which concerns a way of life and well-being at least as much as it does a sharp mind may strike some as far from compelling. Whilst it might be agreed that the reasons for wanting to outline such virtue can be understood, maybe even sympathised with, perhaps they are just as misguided as the metaphysical and ethical realism which they seem to entail.[1] If this wisdom, with its conjunction of practical and theoretical, consists in an awareness of and participation in truth, if it is a kind of knowledge primarily concerned with how we should live, then what place can it have in robust contemporary thinking?[2]

If one individual is to have more knowledge of moral truths than another then there must be moral truths independent of both individuals which they can know. More than this, this wisdom is something which is practised, not merely possessed, so some kind of freedom of volition also seems bound up with this model of virtue. Certainly, Aristotle's treatment merges into a collection of virtues which need not be the direct result of an individual's power, but the core of these virtues, even with Aristotle, concerns a volition (ἡ προαίρεσις; *EN*, §X, viii; 1178ᵃ35), a culpable, unfettered agency which is possessed of a kind of 'self-sufficiency' (ἡ αὐτάρκεια; *EN*, §X, vii; 1177ᵃ25). It is popularly imagined that the problem of determinism and free will was first raised by Epicurus, but as Susanne Bobzien explains, even Epicurus seems to fit more comfortably into an ancient tradition of not recognizing a problem at all (Bobzien 2000, pp. 336–337). Perhaps, as Bobzien suggests, the ancients preferred an attribution of responsibility on the basis of causal origin as opposed to freedom of the will, but it seems safe to say (whilst allowing for exegetical nuances) that along with the metaphysical and ethical realism entailed by this theory of wisdom comes to a quite bold image of the agent as a determiner.

Why does all of this matter anyway? If we are willing to throw away Aristotle's simplistic psychology and Plato's extreme idealism, not to mention the intellectualism that comes with both, why not just discard the naïve realism to boot? Can't we make good use of an idea of wisdom which doesn't involve a world of moral absolutes and mysterious little unmoved movers? Perhaps the most obvious point to make here is that it is hard to say what a virtue concerned with the awareness of and participation in truth would be if there were no such strong idea of truth to engage with. Perhaps it would be concerned with limited truths; perhaps the truths of a community, or (as aforementioned) a species. Human wisdom would be an awareness of and participation in 'human truths'. Ultimately, to deal with this issue comprehensively it would be necessary to treat the myriad arguments for and against relativism and what follows would become little more than a history of those arguments. There are, however, only two primary arguments which will be offered against a relativist objection to this theory of wisdom.

The first argument suggests that ethical relativism is inextricably bound up with a more far-reaching relativism and that any such epistemology will necessarily result in incoherence (which will also be discussed in terms of dishonesty), nihilism or a kind of naïve isolation of volition. This argument will take Nietzsche's discussion of the same topic in *Beyond Good and Evil* as a point both of agreement and departure (Nietzsche 1886, pp. 513–690). This first argument ultimately concludes that any ethical anti-realism will be born out of a fruitless and misplaced desire for certainty which might be dissolved by abandoning a false dichotomy between credulity and incredulity.

The second argument will seek to address an objection to moral realism which might be offered by linguistic philosophy, namely: that ethical talk is meaningless. This argument will suggest that far from ethical language being necessarily meaningless, it is any language which purports to escape this way of talking which will ultimately be meaningless. This argument will take Wittgenstein's identification of both ethics and logic as transcendental structures of our world of meaning as a point of both agreement and departure. Ultimately, this argument will conclude that whilst 'goodness' and 'badness' provide distinct difficulties, 'good things' and 'bad things' *(and the differences therein)* can (and must) be discussed. It will be suggested that any identification of ethical talk as meaningless will rely upon a false dichotomy between ethical and non-ethical ways of life/meaning. The corollary will follow that it is also nonsense to posit any world which is not the ethical-logical one in which we live and that this might also address some of the anti-metaphysical objections of the relativist.

This discussion will then conclude by looking to the more particular problem of free will and determinism which, though not raised directly by the theory of wisdom suggested here, is nevertheless implied. It will be suggested that rather than seeking to wrestle with the twists and turns of apparently irreconcilable inclinations to both freedom and causality, it is possible instead to embrace the spirit of humility and tentative realism hitherto alluded to. Instead of an exhaustive appraisal of compatibilist and incompatibilist theories, an attempt is made to *describe a manner of seeking wisdom which allows some level of intellectual tension and inexplicability to enter into our thinking.* To the linguistic argument for moral realism will be added a kind of attitude or approach inspired by certain aspects of Zen Buddhism; a way of thinking which might allow for navigation of the difficulties of realism without needing to treat the extant points for and against relativism *exhaustively.* An attitude which entails a simple, even naïve belief in the world, moral and physical, as it presents itself, yet one which involves retention of rational enquiry which disallows for a complete victory of this naivety. This view holds all truths, all natures as interdependent. Man is indeed the measure of all things, but so too are all things the measure of Man. That there is a point between stark, clear-cut categories and complete, empty dissolution; that there is a middle path to tread and that this is best;

neither wholly yes, nor wholly no. This middle ground will feed not only into this metaethical theory but also the discussion as a whole.

Between good and evil

Let's imagine philosophy without an ethical or practical basis; intellectual endeavour without ego. Perhaps it would be a logical exercise, an attempt to outline what makes sense and what doesn't. It would be a purely conceptual analysis; let's try to imagine just that, an airy juggling of thoughts, just floating there in an ethereal structure of logic and codified grammar. It might yield truth, such an activity might bear the crisp rationalist fruit of certainty. Unencumbered by the vagaries of life, of observation and experience, this pristine intellectual quest could grant us something immutable. That might be nice. If such a thing were even a possibility, wouldn't it be worth trying? Such cleanliness and clarity. Well, if so, why?

Perhaps just because we like neat things, things which don't rot and change, that might be reason enough to attempt such a practice a priori. We could try an emotivist justification like this, that philosophy, of the conceptual, a priori variety, is simply something which is enjoyed by certain sorts of people, by neat freaks. Such a position would need to deal with the dissonance inherent in a profession of pursuing universal truths whilst attempting to remain content that the desire to do so is based in something so petty, insular, mutable and organic as a personal penchant. To find such a position compelling we would need to embrace, at the very least, an emotional kind of inconsistency, if not a rational one. Or perhaps this philosophy would claim something less grand, not that it seeks truth, but *clarification*. Even here, though, as Wittgenstein acknowledges, there would need to be an ethical axiom which drove us to clarity, some disdain for muddled conversations.[3] It might merely be a therapy for the headaches of metaphysics and other mixed-up language games.[4] It would be a sad little philosophy, though, which took the form of solitary diaries, spelling out purely personal grammatical confusions, thinking nothing for the confusions of others. Perhaps this is what drove Wittgenstein to want to work on a farm instead.[5]

Far more likely, in all of these analytic and linguistic 'philosophies', is a normative suggestion, an ethical stance, however loosely wrought, that to seek the truth, or to remove headaches, is an admirable activity. Of course, such a stance needn't discount the possibility of more visceral, emotive compulsions (and this acknowledgement will be important for what follows). It is being suggested here, however, that some kind of normative basis for a philosophical endeavour (however that activity might be conceived), is not only empirically broadly extant (if not logically necessary), it can also be accurate and hugely compelling.

It is understandable, of course, that someone concerned with the pursuit of truth would want to get as far from emotive and normative motivations as possible. The emotive possibility would, as aforementioned, lead us into a realm of fragile subjectivism of just the sort we neat-minded truth questers hoped to escape. The normative foundation would open a can of ethical worms which cannot help but lead us into the fuzzy dominion of personal experience and uncertainty which we similarly sought to distance ourselves from. Such fears, though, begin to smack of wayward pride.

Nietzsche recognises that any pursuit of truth must necessarily be bound up with a kind of moral quest; he suggests that we can either trust naïvely, blindly even, in these moral and metaphysical truths and thus remain enslaved to our ethical mess, or that we can cast off that inherited paradigm (Nietzsche 1886, §10). Further to this, Nietzsche proposes that the latter option needn't lead to nihilism as we might suspect, in rejecting the fragility of our ethical lives and the pompous pseudo-objectivity of truth-seeking, we needn't crumble into inhuman extinction, rather we (or those strong enough) can and must build ourselves anew; an effulgent, superhuman construct (*Ibid.*). Perhaps this artifice could dissolve any need for the pursuit of wisdom hitherto described.

> The belief in 'immediate certainties' is a moral naïveté which does honour to us philosophers; but – we have now to cease being 'merely moral' men! Apart from morality, such belief is a folly which does little honour to us!... Need I say expressly after all this that they will be free, very free spirits, these philosophers of the future – as certainly they will also not be merely free spirits, but something more, higher, greater, and fundamentally different...
>
> (Nietzsche 1886, §34, 44)

It would be too simple, and quite unfair, to criticise Nietzsche for employing evaluative language in describing his post-moral ideal. Yet it is still hard to say what this elevation of will to the first principle achieves. Certainly, Nietzsche *likes* this overarching drive to manipulate, to change, this 'Will to Power', he approves of it. It is an ethic of preference and escape. Nietzsche has followed the winding path of abstract speculation and he resents the false dichotomy with which he has been presented: accept naiveté and cartoonish truths or relinquish all understanding (so demands the cosmos), and Mr Nietzsche shouts back: No! I shall carve out something else for myself and those who follow me. Nietzsche sees honour in the history of an occupation which has been gripped by a desire for solid, potent truths but urgently proclaims its new mission of *creation*. And he is right, of course, that it is a desire for control, for the safety of a quantity which is known, which drives both he and the truth seeker. But in resolving one false dichotomy, he has ignored other, more subtle options. A gentler path.

The petty dishonesty of the truth seeker who feigns ignorance of the axioms and ethical foundations of her quest; the feeble-mindedness of the non-philosopher who doesn't even start down the path; the pitiful weakness and dissolution of the nihilist who turns away from it all; or the brave new world of the new philosopher as a creator. It is fitting, and not beyond Nietzsche's understanding, that this line-up is itself a fiction. If it is unbearably credulous to believe in truth and justice, then it is at least equally so to believe in any of these strange caricatures. Where is this sea of mindless slaves who wallow perpetually in ignorance and inertia? And what of the nihilist? That gothic, zombie-like ascetic who has failed to pick up her own pieces? Least plausible of all, the superman, the artist extraordinaire, who would need to be so utterly psychologically removed from anything we know that it is barely imaginable, let alone human.[6] Nietzsche's most important gloss, though, is with the truth seeker. Indeed, the dichotomy we are now presented with is between two groups. On the one side are the slaves and the false philosophers, the credulous, and on the other, we have the nihilists and the new philosophers, the incredulous. Belief or doubt. But why not have both?

Does the lover of wisdom necessarily betray her cause when she has faith in truth or goodness? Need this faith be blind? Though a foundation, need it lie there alone and hidden?

Pure, alien, compulsive will remain true, not to the pursuit of truth but to the desire for the safety of certainty. We cannot achieve such certainty through speculation, or through experience, so we can only achieve it by making it ourselves. But why should we take this desire for control and safety to be our bedrock? Is it so self-evidently fundamental to being? Rather, it is suggested here, that the fragile, complex, uncertain ethical realities of life are the irreducible axioms upon which we should build our thought and our lives. Yes, they require some faith, some uncertainty; to accept them as the basis of our thinking requires that we relinquish some aspect of that quest for truth but we needn't give up so much, just the unassailable safety of certainty or the prospect thereof. *It is not a Will to Power which is fundamental to being but meekness.*

Such a loss of certainty need not, however, require a loss of conviction. Certainly, the seeker of wisdom would be giving something precious up if belief and doubt were mutually exclusive. The trap is to think that accepting truth demands unthinking compliance. If I am confident that selfless generosity is a fundamental constituent of the universe and a sound (though not solitary) basis for all of my activity (practical or intellectual), I needn't be a two-dimensional acolyte, hopelessly constrained to accept any and all which bears the mark of such a virtue. Nietzsche himself, of course, was not two-dimensional in his escape:

> There is far too much witchery and sugar in the sentiments 'for others' and 'not for myself'... Let us therefore be cautious!... There is something ticklish in 'the truth' and in the <u>search</u> for truth; and if man goes about it too humanely – 'il ne cherche le vrai que pour faire le bien' – I wager he finds nothing!
>
> (Nietzsche 1886, §33, 35)

Nothing? Yes, let's be *cautious*, yes there can indeed be 'too much witchery and sugar', but need we do this 'too humanely'? Perhaps, just humanely enough might permit us to find something, however small and fragile that something might be. Something in between: not black or white, nor good or evil, nor right or wrong, not knowledge or ignorance, but something in between. Belief and doubt in a complex world of admixture and grey combinations.

Uncertainty

The old philosopher may yet be unconvinced by this call to virtue, however mitigated by claims of moderation. Perhaps there is an option which fuses the nihilist and the truth-seeker: *the sense seeker*. Granted, we do, in practice, employ ethical foundations in all of our dealings, particularly in our 'philosophical' activities. Such things might be unavoidable to an extent, but does that mean we need to engage with them at all times and in all our activities? Can't we just limit our philosophy to avoid such topics, to areas where neatness is possible?

One might even go so far as to say that ethical discourse isn't just messy, it's necessarily nonsensical. Indeed, in his *Lecture on Ethics* Wittgenstein contends just this, transforming Hume's is/ought distinction into a matter of simile and semantic dissonance (Wittgenstein 1929, pp. 9–10). We are told that 'Ethics, if it is anything, is supernatural and our words will only express facts; as a teacup will only hold a teacup full of water and if I were to pour out a gallon over it' (*Ibid.*, p. 7). Thus any attempt at expressing non-instrumental value will necessarily draw upon our language of instrumental value because that's the only kind of value to which we can definitively point, anything else will just overflow into meaninglessness. So when it comes to ethical talk, if we strip away the simile (unlike other occasions of similarity) we are left with nothing (*Ibid.*, p. 9). We may all wish to talk about this empty core to our ethical talk, but we cannot, it is the impenetrable bedrock of our language and necessarily cannot be meaningful: 'running against the walls of our cage is perfectly, absolutely hopeless' (*Ibid.*, p. 12).

But is that what saying something is morally bad or good is really like? When I say, 'she is a bad person' and I am asked 'why do you think she is a bad person?' I might answer by saying that 'she is cruel', I might even give some example of her cruelty. There is certainly a meaning which is being successfully communicated here, and it is not just simply analogous to saying that 'she is bad at tennis'. Attempting to describe *goodness* might be hopeless, attempting to describe *something which is good* and something which is not is certainly not.

Of course, Wittgenstein went on to develop his ideas in new directions. Burbules and Smeyer are right when they identify the reason for Wittgenstein not including more ethical examples of language games as being because ethics is the 'practice of practices' (Burbules and Smeyers 2003, §III). Wittgenstein never departed from his consideration of ethics, aesthetics and other religio-metaphysical matters as being beyond our ability to talk about meaningfully (though he did not dispute their vital importance in our lives) (Wittgenstein 1929, p. 12).[7] Ethical talk is, by this view, a 'tendency in the human mind' (*Ibid.*), a psychological quirk or anthropological curiosity. However foundational or inescapable, it is a habit to be observed rather than a habit of observation.

Now, there are two things which can be said of this model of ethical language which are entirely compatible with the realist theory of wisdom suggested previously and which are most urgent in the demands of relativism. Firstly, (A) it could be said that only people (persons) engage in ethical talk or behaviour and that without people, there would be no right or wrong. Secondly, (B) that ethical truths can only be demonstrated through practice, or by living a certain way of life. Neither of these suggestions precludes the possibility of the reality of ethical truths (the truth conditions of moral facts) independent of the *opinions* of persons.

Before examining in greater detail how these things (A and B) are compatible with a realist understanding of value, it might also be fruitful to consider how they can also be said of logic. 'Logic is not a body of doctrine, but a mirror-image of the world. Logic is transcendental... It is clear that Ethics cannot be put into words. Ethics is transcendental...' (Wittgenstein 1921, §6.13, 6.421). Wittgenstein recognises the similarity; it is just that he prioritises logic as the foundation of that which philosophers should, by his reckoning, be dealing with: language. Certainly, one might be so sceptical so as to question the reality of logical rules beyond the minds of those who use language, but what would such an objection amount to? It would be an empty suggestion, it would rely upon the very thing which it aims to undermine. 'Doubt gradually loses its sense. This language game just *is* like that. And everything descriptive of a language game is part of logic' (Wittgenstein 1969, §56). It would be meaningless to articulate a justification of the rules which govern our ability to convey meaning through language, and yes, any attempt to express or argue for the nature of goodness or badness would be equally vacuous. If there were someone who had no understanding or sense of value whatsoever there would be nothing anyone could explicitly say to enlighten them as to its character. What is argued here though, is that there could, of necessity, be no such '*person*'.

That moral facts are evidently perceived (or conceived of, as the contrary would have it) through quite specific and disparate ways of life (B) leads, quite naturally, to the suspicion that such truths are conventional constructions: fictions which arise out of cultural and psychological pressures. That someone in another time or place could think slavery morally acceptable and that in my own society such a notion seems self-evidently abhorrent might lead people to suspect these opinions to be just that: δόξα; nothing more than the fragile, deluded musings of humanity. But this view, if it is to be anything other than the angry ramblings of the nihilist, if it is to capture the imagination of the philosopher escaping Nietzsche's brave new world, must be cast in the context of how we talk, how we mean and how we live.

Why, we may ask, should the dependence of a way of thinking upon a way of life be restricted to evaluative ways of thinking? Peter Winch, following Wittgenstein's discussions of the dependence of language and thought upon a way of life, set his sights upon the way in which cultural relativism must apply equally to the worlds of scientific and evaluative discourse (Winch 1959–1960 p. 238). When the question becomes 'what do you mean?', reference must be given to the context of communication, the whole world (way of life) out of which has sprung the pronouncement. Before and after, cause and consequence, together and apart, significant and accidental: such seemingly solid, dependable, absolute and mind-independent facts can only be comprehended, only be talked about because we are creatures which live *with* them and *in* them. Living in the world is prior to (or coextensive with) how we talk, how we mean and what we think is important. Pointing out that an appreciation of value(s) is dependent upon living a life (B) tells us nothing since *all* understanding is so dependent.[8]

It is not enough to say that logic and value are the foundations of the way in which *we* live in the world, such a suggestion intimates a duality between persons and some other beyond which can have no meaning. There is simply no point to describing the transcendent horizon which bounds us all as an internally determined Kantian ideal, far less a biological condition. Logic and value are not just how *we* live but how *the world* lives. To describe the way in which our thoughts and language are inseparable from our way of life is not to undermine any possible confidence in the security and reliability of evaluative discourse, instead, it is to dissuade any pretence to epistemological purity whatsoever. To say that all possible meaning is necessarily bound up with being who we are in the world in which we live does not preclude meaningful logical or evaluative assessment, it merely indicates the fallacy of attempting to impose a dualism between unreliable people on the one hand and infallible science and logic on the other.

These kinds of sweeping statements regarding the nature of our world smack of careless, antiquated metaphysics, the sort of thinking characterised by anthropocentrism and a cloying kind of arrogance. Indeed, it would hardly seem possible to square such a world-view with the idea that people are the only kind of moral things in the universe (A); how could such a thing be possible if the universe itself were somehow bound up with the possibility of meaningful value?

The cultural relativist objects that any framework of meaning, any 'world' as is spoken of here, is exclusive to the specific group of people who construct it through their living within it. People and the world are coextensive but private, and there are many such worlds. The biological relativist recognises the horror and absurdity of describing insoluble and incommunicable ethical differences between groups of people; they see that it is apparent that people can and do communicate successfully with one another despite very different ways of life and that to imagine there is some sort of vital cut-off point between cultures is arbitrary and false.[9] To step beyond this biological relativism, to imagine instead that to be *a living thing with a purpose* (with intentions and motivations) is necessary to live in a world of value, is not to suggest that these beings impose this value upon the world, but to describe the way in which both beings and world exist. *A world is such a thing that if it is to be a world in which beings (for which things matter) live, it must be a world in which statements (or beliefs) of a moral nature can be true or false.* Any other kind of world will necessarily be meaningless and will sit within the emptiness of those transcendent edges which define the world in which we do indeed live. We could call this 'universal biological relativism' but it isn't altogether clear why it should be called 'relativism' at all; it will get other names before we are through.

So, it might be plausible to suggest a kind of realism (or universal relativism) based on the way our possibilities of meaning are inextricably bound up with our lives and our world, but what would such a stance amount to? The central and abiding charge against moral realism is, quite rightly, that of arrogance: of 'witchery and sugar'; of unjustifiable confidence. By pointing out the way in which we can mean things, some justification can be offered, not for an assertion of this or that evil or for this or that good, but rather for the kind of knowledge, the kind of factness, that moral facts might represent. δόξα needn't be a *mere* opinion. Exactly how this 'knowledge' might be arrived at, and with what degree of certainty any moral statement might be made is not yet dealt with, only that an escape from the dishonest suspension of disbelief called for by the non-cognitivist is justified. As David Wiggins says:

> ...the non-cognitive account depends for its whole plausibility upon abandoning at the level of theory the inner perspective that it commends as the only possible perspective upon life's meaning. This is a kind of incoherence, and one that casts some doubt upon the distinction of the inside and the outside viewpoints. I also believe that, once we break down the supposed distinction between the inner or participative and the outer, supposedly objective viewpoints, there will be a route by which we can advance (though not to anything like the particularity of the moral certainty that we began by envying).
>
> (Wiggins 1988, p. 135)

This epistemological foundation to a theory of wisdom is 'a route by which we can advance'. Granted, to say that: 'a world is such a thing that if it is to be a world in which beings (for which things matter) live it must be a world in which statements (and beliefs) of a moral nature can be true or false' sounds a bit strong, but it does not mean that moral statements will ever be precisely *true* or *false*, only *more or less true or false*, that judgements about their accuracy can be meaningful. Of course, it is also being suggested, or implied, that people can, by some means, recognise (to some degree of accuracy at least) which moral statement is more true and which more false and act upon this accordingly.

Not one and not two

How is it that we recognise good things and bad things, and, how is it that we act upon that recognition? An indication has already been given as to how we might approach the first of these questions, namely with *a certain moderation in our conviction* (which is to say nothing of the means by which we achieve accuracy, only that we should not expect precision or at least only profess it with a deal of humility and circumspection). Very little has been said regarding our moral powers. Obviously, some sort of position needs to be adopted in relation to both of these questions if the 'realism' hitherto suggested is to be anything other than a matter of mere in important in our understanding of moral intellectual curiosity (which would be an untimely and incongruous termination to such a practically motivated theory). Despite the interconnectedness of these issues, it is the matter of agency and freedom of will which will be most helpful in reaching a conclusion to the moral realism which has been discussed here and which will be the focus of what follows.

Iris Murdoch suggests that:

> As moral agents we have to try to see justly, to overcome prejudice, to avoid temptation, to control and curb imagination, to direct reflection. Man is not a combination of an impersonal rational thinker and a personal will. He is a unified being who sees, and who desires in accordance with what he sees, and has some continual slight control over the direction and focus of his vision.
>
> (Murdoch 1974, p. 40)

Murdoch was combating a climate of moral speculation which sought to draw the conversation ever more in the direction of the naked will, of consideration of a moral being as a moving, dynamic thing rather than a perceiver (*Ibid.*, pp. 1–6).[10] We might forgive, then, those times when Murdoch appears to proclaim perception almost to the total exclusion of will, but we needn't relinquish totally the powers of agency, nor should we. Murdoch's summary, however much as it might favour perception, aptly highlights *the inextricable link between recognising what is good and trying to do what is good.* The arena of this 'trying', this agency, might well be dwarfed by the immensity of the mechanical storm which sweeps us through existence, but however salutary an understanding of this diminution might be, we suspect that autonomy must play some part in goodness. Moral realism requires some 'continual slight control'; whether this is simply over the direction of our attention or over other sorts of actions is (at this juncture) relatively unimportant, the exertion of a (partially) self-determined energy is the same.

The temptation is to become metaphysical in our speculations. The world of causes and consequences, especially viewed through the lens of a scientific age, would seem to disallow for any of these magical properties and spontaneous (it might even be said arbitrary) psychological activities. Even if we were inclined to allow for the less tangible phenomenon of free will, the law of non-contradiction, the core of logic itself, presses our ideas into a deadly conflict. Either we are free or we are determined. Our tandem inclinations, to believe in both material, causal universe and true moral responsibility, appear to be in a doomed relationship, from which only one may emerge intact.

Various arguments might be made for the compatibility of these conflicting inclinations, frequently taking the form of a kind of psychological assessment, leaving intact causal determination and instead seeking to demonstrate what is really important in our understanding of moral responsibility.[11]

A Perhaps the end results of our actions are unavoidable. We might use Frankfurt's example of a murder with a backup plan.[12] If the murderer hadn't committed the act voluntarily, the backup plan would have ensured that the murder took place. So the sequence of events in the universe may be unalterable but what matters for moral responsibility are the intentions of agents. We think someone guilty even if they cannot change what happens in the end.

B Perhaps instead we might say that a person who cannot help but be good is still a good person and vice versa. So a hero who saves some innocent people trapped in a burning building who later explains that she couldn't have done otherwise might be telling the truth and we would still think them a hero (maybe even more so).

C Perhaps a moral agent simply needs to be responsive to the right sorts of reasons. So, again, a creature whose actions are determined by the right sorts of causes is the sort of creature upon which moral responsibility can appropriately be heaped. A robot or a hypnotised somnambulist are not morally responsible because they aren't responding to the right sorts of causes. Moral responsibility is just a kind of way we treat a certain sort of determined system, one which contains moral reasons as part of its mechanism.[13]

D Or perhaps these reasons need to accord with a second-order desire. So a morally responsible person is the sort who, upon reflection on their own desires, desires to have these desires.[14]

These are the likely sorts of positions which might be turned to in reaction to the conflict between our inclination to apportion moral responsibility and, simultaneously, to believe in a universe where every event is a consequence necessarily preceded by a corresponding cause. It might well be worth considering, if only briefly, that a conviction in such a rigidly causal universe could be shaken by anything from Hume's thoughts on the idea of causation (Hume 1748, §4:1:1–13) to even a cursory understanding of modern physics.[15] But to follow that path any great distance would prove messy, metaphysical and tangential.

In regards to the idea that it is simply intentions which matter, and an 'ability to do otherwise' does not (A), we may well suspect that, despite ultimate eventualities being unimportant in apportioning responsibility, it might still be deemed important that the person has determined, *independently*, their own intentions. This element at least must demonstrate some freedom. As for the person who cannot help but intend good things (B) (perhaps the sort of thing Murdoch is imagining) we might say that, yes they are good, perhaps even a hero, but this is a different sort of good from someone who must make some kind of effort, someone who has some kind of inclination to *not* run into burning buildings. Additionally, we might simply disallow for the alternative being possible. To imagine any person who acts in such a way that every element of their activity is entirely without contrary inclinations, either historically or presently, is not to imagine a person at all. One might jump to someone's aid instantly, and this is good, but it is part of a history of inclination and cultivation, we are moral through our history, not only in an instant.[16]

All of this kind of incompatibilist counter-argumentation is certainly useful for bolstering our reasons for being cautious of the comfort offered by these responsibilities without free-will. We might, however, simply recognise the compelling insight of those compatibilist positions which highlight the role of reasons in our moral thinking (particularly of the type C). We do indeed think of moral behaviour being 'caused' by moral reasons. In this sense, Murdoch seems right to suggest that a good person is the kind of person who sees what is good and *therefore* aims for it.

Of course, it is the 'therefore', the 'cause' of moral reasons which is problematic, and we may well suspect that we are being tempted to think about moral inspiration, reasoning and perception in a way modelled on mechanical and physical causation and that this is to confuse incommensurable ways of thinking, to confuse our language games. We might instead follow Fischer and Ravizza (1993) and attempt to amend our vocabulary and speak instead of a 'responsiveness' to reasons. Or perhaps, like Anscombe (1957) we might review the psychology of intention and willful desire in greater detail and thus attempt to clarify the range of activities and kinds of conversations which might be covered by this idea of moral reasons and 'causation'.

However, much one might attempt to reduce the conflict between determinism and moral responsibility to psychological or metaphysical misconceptions, one's efforts will leave a phenomenological remainder. However much any of these theories of responsibility without freedom might affirm the diminished place of any freedom which we might hope to have, they do not extinguish the pivotal role which some sense of self-determined liberty plays in the reality of our moral lives. Nor does any criticism of the scientific and metaphysical difficulties of causation itself detract from the immediately apparent reality of both mechanical and psychological causation in our lives.

Just as 'a world is such a thing that if it is to be a world in which beings (for which things matter) live it must be a world in which statements (and beliefs) of a moral nature can be true or false' so too does it seem to be one in which these moral statements (and beliefs) can not only be more or less accurate but also one in which they can be 'freely' intended. If good and bad form part of the ineffable boundary which defines our world then free will and determinism occupy a similar realm. Our experience of the freedom of our volition is prior to any speculation about its conflict with causation, and it is concurrent with our experience of that causation. Both causation (moral causation in the form of reasons) and 'free will' suffuse our lived experience in tandem. Together they form part of the basic fabric of life which precedes and shapes any discussion of their ultimate nature.

If there is going to be some double-think, some sleight-of-hand (and seemingly there must be), it must come as part of the muddle, not as a solution to it. Better the tyrant who fails openly in weakness and frailty than the one who fails in secrecy through corruption and lies. Some vices are worse than others. We must remember the courage of Socrates' philosophic soldier. Even the hardest granite wall will crack over time, and though it is the very bedrock, given to us as an impermeable layer beneath which lies only impossibly blinding fire and upon which all else is built, it is itself the very model of all else in the world: it breaks. And though the cracks and weather-beaten recesses might upset those who look for symmetry, cleanliness or permanence, they are of incomparable beauty next to the shallow plaster and whitewash which would cover their roughness.

As with so many philosophical problems the demands of our enquiring inclination, that tidy-minded quest for certainty, conflicts with the vital weight of our common-sense. There is a kind of singularity, conceptually infinitesimal and impenetrable conjunction upon which our basic lived realities hinge; where freedom requires being determined by good reasons and our world of causes and consequences, of persons performing actions, requires agents which self-determine in order to be the universe we recognise every day. It is where the psychological gap between intention and action closes to indistinction. To seek to 'resolve' this conflict under the auspices of the law of contradiction is to expect an infinite regress of logical conformity where none exists. It is, once again, to succumb to a spirit of cleanliness and ambition which is inevitably shaken to pieces when it too reaches beyond its limits.

Perhaps then it is the business of philosophy, though it can do nothing with this ineffable point about which our moral world hinges, to approach this precipice as far as it can and to maintain it as an apophatic point of focus, a reminder and pivot to which our humility, our determination to do good and to seek truth is tethered. To ensure that the wavering and ineffable boundaries are permitted to neither be forgotten nor indulged to the point where they can overwhelm our common sense is the inescapable charge of the enquiring mind. As Zen master Qingyuan explains:

Before I had studied Zen for thirty years, I saw mountains as mountains, and waters as waters. When I arrived at a more intimate knowledge, I came to the point where I saw that mountains are not mountains, and waters are not waters. But now that I have got its very substance I am at rest. For it's just that I see mountains once again as mountains, and waters once again as waters Qingyuan Xingsi.

(n.d./2000, p. 975)

Rather than attempt to reconcile seemingly irreconcilable and contradictory principles, *it may simply be better to describe a possible attitude to adopt in the face of these difficulties*. To imagine that the rigorous demands of logic and the steady measure of rational enquiry are necessarily at odds with the impressions and assumptions which underlie our daily existence is to give credence to the demands of logical enquiry first and foremost. It would, however, be a peculiar thing to describe a moral realist theory of wisdom and take it as an axiom without any attempt at an excuse, it would then be only a small supplement to this to suggest that logic and rational enquiry necessarily fail us and we must soldier on without their aid.

In an effort to escape the punishing rigour of the law of non-contradiction this sort of mystical religiosity would simply set up its own tyrant in the place of another. Instead, perhaps, a spirit of 'semi-dualism' might be employed in order that the squabbling inclinations of our lives can cohabit. Master Qingyuan's Zen quest need not be read as a grand, life-long narrative, but a continuous process. Not an attempt to move from naivety to nihilism and then to naivety again, but rather to move from the two in opposition to both in combination. To hold, at all times, both doubt and conviction in one's mind, a world of both freedom and inevitability, of immediate truths, moral and otherwise, and of deep, impenetrable secrets, this is the principle of not one and not two.[17] Doubtless, there are times and activities where one principle will weigh more heavily than another, but conciliation and admixture, even balance, are not synonymous with homogeneity.

This pseudo-Zen principle may well bring us back to the humility of Socrates. An old man faced with hostility and injustice who rests in the comfort of what he 'knows' to be truly important, and who smiles, both derisively and resignedly at the senseless confusion around him; and so too might the illogical boundaries which the Zen master hovers upon lie most convincingly in a smile. The stubbornness of the universe not to conform to our expectations and desires and the confusion which this engenders might lead to a kind of panic, or despondency, or *it might just make us laugh*. This is not the mindless, empty-eyed smile of nihilism, ascetic transcendence, or bloody-minded faith, nor is it the maniacal grin of a carnival of chaos and lunacy, it is, rather, *the smile of knowing contentment*, of one who searches through the ashes of their burnt home and finds their most precious family heirloom unharmed; a realistic, deeply contextualised hopefulness and gratitude.

Indeed it is not a *theory* of free will or certainty, nor of moral realism which it is important to take forward into this enquiry of wisdom, instead, it is this *attitude* of good-humoured understanding in the face of overwhelming conceptual and moral conflicts at the heart of our lives. It is this attitude which will be crucial throughout this discussion.

In many ways this theory of realism closely follows that expressed (at times) by G. K. Chesterton in his 'Orthodoxy'. Chesterton too associates his realism with a kind of common sense of sanity or soundness of mind, one which is anchored in an attitude to a contradiction. He explains how:

> The ordinary man has always been sane because the ordinary man has always been a mystic. He has permitted the twilight. He has always had one foot in earth and the other in fairyland. He has always left himself free to doubt his gods; but (unlike the agnostic of to-day) free also to believe in them... Thus he has always believed there was such a thing as fate, but such a thing as free will also...It is exactly this balance of apparent contradictions which has been the whole buoyancy of the healthy man. The whole secret of mysticism is this: that man can understand everything by the help of what he does not understand.
>
> (Chesterton 1908, p. 35)

This talk of mysticism and fairyland may cause us to suspect, like Nietzsche, the presence of 'too much witchery and sugar'. The proclamations of a Roman Catholic apologist like Chesterton about what we should and should not just accept may well conjure up an air of dogma which sits poorly in any well-formed epistemology, and Chesterton certainly does go on to espouse far more of the belief than he does the doubt. But the spirit of conviction and confusion which Chesterton discusses is not dependent upon the catechism (as much as he might insist it is), nor is it alien to other traditions (as he also suggests). The concept of ἐποχή (epoché), as employed by the 'Hellenistic philosophers' often has much in common with what is being expressed here, and there is a great deal of continuity to be drawn between that concept and the moderate realist attitude being described here (Cooper 2013, pp. 286–287). The two reasons for not using this ancient terminology at this juncture are that (a) ancient use of this term is not univocal and, as such, would require substantial exegesis and (b) that the most plausible reading of ἐποχή is far more like that practised by Chesterton's 'agnostic'; a suspension of judgement. For example, when Sextus Empiricus suggests that:

> ...rather, since the Dogmatists seem plausibly to have established that there is a standard of truth, we have set up plausible-seeming arguments in opposition to them, affirming neither that they are true nor that they are more plausible than those on the contrary side, but concluding to suspension of judgement because of the apparently equal plausibility of these arguments...
>
> (Sextus Empiricus, *Outlines of Pyrrhonism*, 2:79)

We get the sense very much of rational intellectual disengagement. Yet both this sceptical suspension of judgement and Chesterton's epistemology and ethics (with all its accepted impenetrability, mysticism and hiddenness) share some psychology in common and do reflect part of the attitude being enquired into here.

Ultimately the question as to where to draw the line as to just how much of this cloud of unknowing can play a part in our thoughts is a complex one. Chesterton is certainly correct when he indicates that solid and unquestioned conviction in certain truths is a necessary part of a healthy and correct attitude, though we may suspect that his division of humility into that which lies in the 'organ of conviction' and that in the 'organ of ambition' may be too simplistic (Chesterton 1908, p. 41). We cannot simply doubt ourselves and not our other convictions.

It has already been suggested that the ambition and pride behind a desire for endless order, comprehension and cohesion are at the heart of much of the psychology of a certain kind of philosophy. Although we can recognise what Chesterton seeks to achieve by dividing belief in one's self from belief in other things, and apportioning massive doubt to one and little or none to the other, we can also recognise the continuity between the two. When I am humble about my own abilities I cannot so easily exclude my powers of reasoning or of sensation from that humility. This is not to deny, of course, that certain things, frequently those more tangible experiences, are less susceptible to the doubts raised as part of this humility, but doubt and humility are not synonymous. Wittgenstein is correct that certain doubts, when expressed, simply make no sense, but this doesn't prevent a much broader kind of tentative attitude towards one's enquiries, however cerebral or otherwise these might be. One can be humble without rigorously doubting anything and everything. A line must be drawn.

How and where these lines should be drawn is the topic of what follows. Of course, such a broad mission statement might be taken as a definition of ethics itself, but it is by means of a moderate realist attitude that this current line-drawing activity shall be conducted. Indeed, the enquiry which follows into the nature of wisdom and how it can be employed in our lives is both built upon and offered in support of this 'balance of apparent contradictions'. This theoretical and psychological balance is the principle in the light of which ideas of wisdom and wellbeing will be measured. Harmony or balance does not necessitate monotony or homogeneity; complex admixtures with apparent extremes, and even imperfections, can form balanced wholes. Just as the sculptures which once adorned the Parthenon express fine detail, elegant form, realist mayhem, harmonious proportion, the scars of time and poignant imperfections, so too can wisdom and wellbeing consist of many complex and interwoven elements. Our lives, of love and making do, of success and failure, these lives are expressions of this attempt at balance and, as Aristotle suggests, are the crucial test to which we must turn our enquiries.

Notes

1 I am thinking here mostly of a kind of non-cognitivism which I regularly, even routinely encounter (what Russ Shafer-Landau calls 'expressivist' [Shafer-Landau 2005, pp. 19–22]). Usually, my own moral realist stance will provoke a kind of indignance coupled with the suggestion that moral language simply isn't of the fact claiming kind, which, as for reasons that will become clear, I find to be a curiously weak and empirically flawed objection.

2 In addition to Shafer-Landau, it is now gratifying to be able to count the work of Derek Parfit (2017). In the final volume of Parfit's *On What Matters*, he offers the hitherto embattled and forsaken ranks of moral realism a high profile and robust champion. As will be seen, the realism suggested here is of a different kind to the non-naturalism of Parfit and Shafer Landau, but it shares with them much fundamental dissatisfaction with the relativist status-quo.

3 I am thinking here particularly of the section of the *Philosophical Investigations* where Wittgenstein almost seems to pause and asks: 'Where does our investigation get its importance from, since it seems only to destroy everything interesting, that is, all that is great and important? (As it were all the buildings, leaving behind only bits of stone and rubble.) What we are destroying is nothing but houses of cards and we are clearing up the ground of language on which they stood' (L. Wittgenstein 1953, §118). I don't read Wittgenstein's first question as entirely rhetorical. The 'clearing up' which comes as a triumphant answer here cannot help but seem a little lacklustre. Who but the most terminally, obsessively, compulsive would accept such a replacement for 'all that is great and important'?

4 Rather than explicitly throwing my pennyworth into the arena of Wittgensteinian exegesis and the Theory vs Therapy debate, I hope instead that my own discussion of the counter-productive attempt to separate clear thinking and good living will offer a less obviously partisan contribution. I suspect that my own disdain for solid and easy to wield answers (theories) fits particularly well with a reading of Wittgenstein which focuses on an attempt to draw philosophy away from ideas of progress and, as such, finds some sympathy with Daniel Hutto's 'third way' (Hutto 2003, p. 5).

5 On Wittgenstein's efforts to elope to the USSR see: R. Monk's (1990, pp. 151–152) *Ludwig Wittgenstein: The Duty of Genius*.

6 I agree with Keith Ansell-Pearson that 'Nietzsche does not intend Zarathustra to teach something utterly fantastical' (Ansell-Pearson 1992, p. 317). I do not mean 'unimaginable' or 'inhuman' in a dramatic sense, but rather in a sense of psychological naivety and two-dimensional, implausibility. I agree also with Ansell-Pearson that the basis of this 'overman' is in a kind of personal progress (we might say 'overcoming'), and for this reason, this current discussion finds great sympathy with Nietzsche's quest. But Nietzsche's answer is to reduce the human to a kind of minimalist impulse, empty of moral intuition. My challenge is not, as with those against whom Ansell-Pearson takes issue, with Nietzsche's logical problems (as will become clear[er], that would be somewhat hypocritical) but with the almost foetal, creative core which Nietzsche identifies as vital, desirable and, in some sense, attainable. In place of Nietzsche's self-immolation and rebirth, I attempt to suggest a gentler compromise, or perhaps the occasional self-beratement.

7 Wittgenstein concludes his lecture by emphasising his enduring respect for ethical talk.

8 Winch (1967, p. 112) can certainly be read as suggesting a kind of relativism. Alisdair MacIntyre reads Winch in this way when he complains that a cultural determination of all thought would preclude the possibility of change: '...on

Winch's view certain actual historical transitions are made unintelligible...'. Though it might also be suggested that, given his focus on 'intelligibility' such a position would be unintelligible (This is the position taken by W. P. Brandon [1982, p. 21] in *'Fact' and 'Value' in the Thought of Peter Winch: Linguistic Analysis Broaches Metaphysical Questions*).

9 At this point, it is important to note that there is no working consensus on just what does and does not count as 'cultural relativism'. 'Biological relativism' (as I call it here) of the sort expressed by the likes of Martha Nussbaum (perhaps articulated most comprehensively in *Creating Capabilities*, (2011, pp. 110–111) seems entirely compatible with the kind of 'cultural relativism 2.0' described by Michael Brown in *Cultural Relativism 2.0* (2008, pp. 363–383). Brown insists that the discipline of anthropology is not so riddled with Boazian relativism as is often claimed and suggests that a kind of relativism which far more closely resembles the 'moderate realism' expressed in this current discussion is more representative of what is genuinely believed. I hope Brown is correct about this.

10 An understanding of ethics as primarily a matter of perception (or at least in addition to 'reason') is important throughout this book. Murdoch is important in this regard and towards the close of the book, I turn more to Weil's idea of 'attention'. Of great importance in forming these ideas has been the work of Michael Hauskeller (see particularly: Hauskeller's *The Relation between Ethics and Aesthetics in Connection with Moral Judgements about Gene Technology* (2002, pp. 99–102)). Hauskeller recognises the close relationship between evaluative judgements and the kind of visceral observations which we might more happily associate with aesthetics.

11 I am talking here primarily about the compatibilism of Strawson (1962, pp. 45–66), Wolf (Wolf 1981, pp. 101–118), Frankfurt (Frankfurt 1969, pp. 829–839), and Fischer and Ravizza (1993, pp. 1–44).

12 Otherwise known as 'Frankfurt Cases' (Frankfurt, 1969).

13 This is the view defended by Fischer and Ravizza (1993, pp. 31–33) as they describe in the introduction to *Perspectives on Moral Responsibility*.

14 Frankfurt makes this condition of second-order desire a necessary part of personhood; he calls those creatures without these desires 'wantons'. This will be of some relevance later in this discussion (Frankfurt 1971, pp. 5–20).

15 On the idea of causation and quantum physics see Roland Omnés' (2002, particularly pp. 69–71) *Quantum Philosophy* in which Omnés appeals directly to Hume's epistemology.

16 It is important to note at this juncture the role played by Elizabeth Anscombe (1958) in shaping this return to Aristotle and an ethics based on the idea of cultivating a moral character over time. See particularly: *Modern Moral Philosophy*, in *Philsosophy*.

17 Such a reading of the pure land tradition is not without precedent, as discussed by E. McCarthy (2011, p. 225) in *Beyond the Binary: Watsuji Tetsuro and Luce Irigaray on Body, Self and Ethics*.

4 An amalgamation of philosophy and anthropology as the best method for gaining wisdom

More Things in Heaven and Earth.

(Shakespeare, *Hamlet*, 1.5)

What's this then? This book right here, right now, what is it about? It's all well and good describing a grand affirmation of an attitude of moderate moral realism and pseudo-Zen non-dualistic good-humour, but what does that mean for an investigation into wisdom? And what good could such an investigation achieve anyway? Certainly, something has already been said about wisdom. That it should be a pervasive and fundamental thing in life, that it has something to do with an attitude towards who and what we are; not just some cognitive attitude but something enacted, something lived. Indeed, it has been suggested that it is something which can be furthered by being practised.

By all accounts then, if this book is to shed any more light on wisdom, to make some substantive claims about this humble and inquisitive way of living, it must, in some sense, be a practical exercise. Of course, there is a very immediate sense in which an exercise in academic philosophy (as this book might be considered) is already an exercise in seeking wisdom. If possessing wisdom consists in understanding better that which is important, and if wisdom itself is something important, and to understand wisdom better one must possess some wisdom, then seeking to understand wisdom better seems like a promising way to become wiser.

If:

1 P is things possessed.
2 I is important things.
3 U is things understood.
4 W is wisdom.

Then:

1 Some P is I.
2 Every U is P.
3 Some U is I – this is W: the intersection of U and I (and P).

And:

1   W (w) is a member of W (the set contains itself).[1]

Helpful? It doesn't seem terribly practical, not for everyday life anyway. Cogitating on the difficulties of one's occupation being the focus of one's occupation is a far cry from the trials and tribulations of day-to-day living (however petty or abstract those maybe). If, though, 'life', in this vague and grand way, is to be the fount and fulcrum of wisdom, certain critical questions must be asked before any further enquiry can be made; namely:

1   Whose 'everyday' is to count as 'everyday'? For an academic, these sorts of abstract problems are 'everyday', for a less than philosophical accountant or lumberjack, probably not so much.
2   Provided some agreeable understanding can be reached as to what counts as 'everyday life', what method can be used to glean the aforementioned wisdom from this life? Is it psychological? Anthropological? Ethological?

The short responses to these two queries are:

1   Everyone's everyday life is everyday life. All forms and walks of life will offer some wisdom, many will offer common insights. Since every aspect of every life is too grand a remit for any enquiry, it will be suggested that some ways of life not only shed light on more wisdom(s), but also that they do so by demonstrating more of what has been discussed already in terms of 'balance' (a *sustainable* holding together of conflicting things) and that these are subsequently suitable foci for this enquiry. The purpose of describing these ways of life in terms of 'everyday' is to highlight both the universality and common nature of the wisdom they employ/reveal, and also to highlight the necessity of academic philosophy to remove itself from its traditional bounds in order to achieve its own goals.
2   Yes it is psychological, anthropological and ethological. It is self-help, it is autoethnography, it is journalism, history, politics, classics, literary criticism, comparative mythology, mythopoesis and theology. It is science, it is art, and it is all of these things because it is *philosophy*.

Of course, these responses raise more questions than they answer, but such is the joy of philosophy.

Disciplinary distinction certainly serves a purpose, and Anthony Kenny seems right when, in the general introduction to his 'History of Western Philosophy', he claims that:

...once problems can be unproblematically stated, when concepts are uncontroversially standardised, and where a consensus emerges for the methodology of solution, then we have a science setting up home independently, rather than a branch of philosophy.

(Kenny 2012, p. xi)

It would be absurd to suggest that at all times every question must be asked explicitly as part of some grand lifelong quest for ultimate truth and meaning, for the fulfilment of one's purpose and sense of wellbeing. We needn't restrict this non-philosophy to the routines of lab or blackboard either; very simple, mundane questions are regularly asked in a 'non-philosophical' way. 'Where did you leave the keys?' for instance, or 'How long until supper is ready?', are excellent examples of questions for which both terms and conditions are well agreed upon and methodologically settled. Controversy darkens not the face of mindless mediocrity and the comfortably run-of-the-mill. At least, not at first glance. But philosophy is always in the second glance.

Though we might agree that there are times, in both science and practical existence, when uncritical assent is both appropriate and desirable, we may yet permit the philosophical eye to hover just beyond the stage as a kind of psychological overseer. This kind of concurrent assent and dissent has already been described in relation to a foundational epistemology and ethical attitude in the previous chapter. So, although genetics might be allowed practical sovereignty over its realm of cells and spirals, its borderlands will always be patrolled by its philosophical sire, its skies populated by invisible ancestors. Philosophy is the parent who never dies, whose estate is never wholly inherited.

So, whilst it is evidently true that many aspects of life, academic disciplines included, are not immediately concerned with the sort of self-improvement and big-picture, ethical scrutiny which characterises wisdom (as hitherto discussed), they may yet be so in an indirect way. Big discoveries are made through lots of little questions.

Consilience

Vogel Carey attributes the coinage of this term to William Whewell (2013). For Whewell, it designated the way in which scientific discoveries can and do agree with one another in unexpected ways and that this agreement is a compelling reason to believe the discovery. E. O. Wilson (1998) commandeers this term and uses it in a somewhat stronger sense; he uses it to describe a kind of unity of scientific knowledge which is at the heart of all science. Whether one allows for Wilson's adaptation, this term refers to something like the unity of knowledge (and virtue) which both Aristotle and Plato suggest and which is at the heart of the theory of wisdom being discussed here. It is also the sort of thing which Masanobu Fukuoka is concerned with when he suggests that:

> Lately I have been thinking that the point must be reached when scientists, politicians, artists, philosophers, men of religion, and all those

who work in the fields should gather here, gaze out over these fields, and talk things over together. I think this is the kind of thing that must happen if people are to see beyond their specialties.

(Fukuoka 1978)

Whether by surprise or design, when blind men put the different parts of the elephant together, they fit. Ultimately it is the elephant which is at the heart of things.

Specialisation has its weaknesses, it drifts away from the big picture, away from context. 'How long until supper is ready?' is certainly a question which it is forgivable, indeed laudable, to ask without too much reflection. But we do ask such questions for a reason. We dine at certain times of the day, eating certain quantities. When supper is ready is dependent upon affluence, free time, historical models of labour, nutrition, health, dedication to quality of food and the commensality of dining experiences. These facts too are related to geographic location and methods of cultivation. Before long one is brought to consider very broad questions of politics and economics, also of the role of diet in social life and physical wellbeing, of the rights of those who have laboured, suffered and died to produce the food. How we eat and where our food comes from are not trivial matters, indeed few matters are quite so significant.

Simplicity and complexity, prevalence and significance; these are not mutually exclusive, they are complimentary

The accountant, the lumberjack, the geneticist, they all get up in the morning and go to work. The accountant is confronted with the records of a friend, the finances of whom are in a shambles, and is faced with the difficult matter of explaining how dire the situation is and how extreme and immediate the changes must be. The lumberjack begins to feel the aches of advancing age, the icy wind bites deeper and the weight of the chainsaw bears more heavily on the knuckles and knees; each day makes more apparent their younger colleagues' superior strength and questions of self-worth are unavoidable. The geneticist, head of their department, is faced with reduced budgets and must discontinue one of their projects; longevity or heart disease, which is the more deserving of study?

It is not only patronising and narrow-minded to imagine that some life, base and crude, is devoid of philosophy, it is also inaccurate and a failure of the quest for insight. The value of the insight offered by the immediate and palpable experience of these dilemmas cannot be overestimated. The classic problem of the undergraduate philosophy seminar, when someone inevitably asks whether it is, in fact, wrong to kill babies, rings hollow when confronted with genuine dilemmas of Ayoreo women wrestling with the demands of family life and broken marriages when they must choose between very great evils.[2]

Of course, it is a shallow and trite suggestion that one cannot possibly understand a topic unless one has had the first-hand experience of the matter. The objection that 'you can't understand this unless you are... X (let's say 'a parent')' is the sort of galling, narrow-minded conversation stopper which I mean. But this kind of claim could be toned down. To say, then, that direct involvement *can* grant a deeper and distinct sort of insight from mere abstraction seems quite reasonable. Indeed, it could quite plausibly be suggested that abstraction and direct experience are complimentary to a fuller understanding. This is, in fact, very much what is being (and will be further) suggested here. The parent has a unique insight, but so too does the incisive, abstract thinker. Wisdom is to be found in the realisation of the contiguity of these sources of insight.

This, then, is the working hypothesis (part one): *that philosophy (a mindful pursuit of [self- and other-] improvement through abstract enquiry, critical thinking and the cultivation of a passion for learning) and the commonplace pursuit of work, wealth, sustenance, wellbeing, family life and wider success engaged in by the vast majority of (at least) human beings are not only compatible but, when 'done properly', mutually beneficial and, ultimately inextricable.*

To test this hypothesis, it will be necessary (or at least appropriate) to take an example of 'daily life done properly' and examine whether or not it does encompass what is being talked about here as philosophy (this pursuit of wisdom).

The examination of 'daily life done properly' will be conducted primarily through a study of permaculture (or what might more generally be thought of as 'organic self-provision gardening'). This will be for (broadly) three reasons:

1 This is a way of life with which I am personally familiar and which I have found not only to be intimately connected with my experience of philosophy but also with a more general sense of wellbeing and perspective which has here been discussed as part of (or identical to) 'wisdom'.
2 It is a practice which is peculiarly rich in its amalgamation of ethical content (social, environmental and virtue) and its engagement with 'life' in a very universal sense. (This ethical 'richness' will be expanded upon below in relation to a general methodology of anthropological philosophy).
3 It is a way of life which, despite the modern guise in which I shall encounter it, is ultimately an expression of the most basic and enduring of activities (encompassing work, diet, family life, prosperity, etc.) and through which our own activities are least removed from those of other 'life'. This 'basic' quality shares much in common with the principles of philosophy.

As David Cooper remarks at the outset of his discussion of *The Philosophy of Gardens*: 'there is no discipline to be introduced' (Cooper 2006, p. 1).

To both Cooper's and my own bemusement gardens have not been treated (in the extant philosophical corpus) with the level of seriousness and diligence which seems intuitively correct. Cooper's treatment of the topic of gardens does, however, diverge significantly from my own approach. It would be fair to say that where Cooper treats 'gardens' I treat the more specific topic of 'permaculture'. There are certain synergies between Cooper's work and this book (particularly at this book's close) and it is only right that an acknowledgement of *A Philosophy of Gardens* should be explicit and emphatic. Cooper does, for instance, explore the relationship between gardening and the cultivation of virtues and it is this topic which is at the core of this book (*Ibid.*, p. 93). As such, I hope that there is some room to conceive of this discussion as an expansion of that one topic of Cooper's introductory work and, whilst it may move in directions which Cooper does not (or would not) entertain, I also hope that it does employ the seriousness which Cooper desires for this topic.

This current study of *permaculture* will be conducted through an admixture of anthropological and philosophical methodologies (as opposed to more conventional conceptual analysis). For reasons expanded upon below, this amalgam will, in fact, be viewed as reflective of a single, more fruitful and appropriate method of enquiry which is commensurate with 'philosophy as a way of life'. Autoethnography, multi-species ethnography and abstract conceptual analysis: these seemingly separate methodologies are an integral part of the conscilience (or 'holism') of this book as a whole.

'Daily life done properly'

This is not a phrase which fits comfortably into many well-thought through conversations. It is a familiar sort of phrase in the field of 'philosophy as a way of life' and various other branches of moral philosophy, nevertheless, it is likely to conjure discomfort elsewhere. By what means will the properness of the doing be judged? Always supposing we can arrive at some idea of 'daily life' which covers enough ways of living so as to be viewed as somehow representative or inclusive. And if some criterion, by which the properness of this doing might be judged, were considered justified, wouldn't that leave the whole process of scrutinising this daily life for evidence of wisdom redundant? If one were to say: 'let's find out what a good life is like by looking at a good life' one would be in the tricky position of needing to know what a good life was like already in order to judge an appropriate subject of study.

Luckily Meno's paradox, of which this is an example, admits to some possible moderation.[3] In this regard, there are two responses to this aporia worth considering. Firstly, we need not have a comprehensive understanding of the properness of the doing in order to have *some reasonable suspicion* that it is being done properly. I can think that someone seems to be doing something well and not have a detailed understanding of how that is so. Secondly, we might be wrong. As long as one has a reasonable suspicion that life is being done properly, as long as one's inspection of that life permits the possibility that it is not being done properly, one's investigation needn't be considered artificial or unacceptably biased.

Of course, still we are left with the criterion by which we judge the *reasonableness of our suspicion* that a life is being lived properly or well. It might be objected that any such suspicion cannot possibly be justified, that there are no values on which to draw which do not already infuse the investigation with an unacceptably high level of personal preference.

Of course, it would be foolish (or at least dull) to be dragged back altogether into a concern over cultural relativism, and just as before it will be maintained that there are indeed certain broad values which are not only common to most 'daily lives', past and present, but which can reasonably form the basis for judging whether or not a life seems to be being lived well. It must also be noted that no claim has been made to the exclusivity of any such life, so some level of personal preference, which might fairly be viewed as inevitable, may yet be considered permissible. In this way, if one were a reindeer herder, and thus had an inclination to look for a well-lived life amongst arctic herders, one might nevertheless concede that fishermen in the western pacific could live quite a different sort of life and still live it well.[4] There can be many forms of life lived well. We may, though, suspect that there will be some common elements between these distant paragons of virtue.

Certainly this idea of common virtues is consistent with the Greek theory of virtue and of wisdom which has formed the point of departure for this discussion. Aristotle says: 'in general, all men seek not the way of their forefathers, but rather, the good' (*Politics*, §2:1269a:1-5).[5] There are common excellences to which we should aspire. So, if we were inclined to be persuaded by this antique vision of virtue, we might look about for rumours of courage, of justice, of temperance and, of course, wisdom. Perhaps, if we felt like permitting our list of virtues to creep closer to our own times we might even allow for some more medieval, Christian flavours, like charity or piety. But need we be so specific? Might not the virtues be more nebulous than this effort to categorise suggests (particularly if they are unified through wisdom as has been said)? Perhaps we might also allow the virtues we seek to be a little less constrained by the context of ancient Athenian gentlemanly conduct or the cloistered order of medieval monasteries.

We have already encountered the mother of large families which Murdoch raises; in that case we can still think of courage, still think of temperance and justice. So it may be fair to identify some very broad ideals as common to all persons and expressed in many diverse (and frequently not very exceptional) circumstances. It is this sense of a unity of virtue which will be taken forward very much in the way Aristotle speaks of 'ἀρετὴ πρὸς τὴν κυρίαν', or 'κυρίως ἀγαθὸν' (*EN*, VI: xiii, 1144b3, 6).[6] Which is not, as has been said, to carry over the stronger Aristotelean commitment to a heavily intellectual epistemic fulcrum, nor the Platonic adherence to an inherent, a priori virtuousness, but rather the sense of an underlying and common thread of goodness which connects all instances of goodness.

How far beyond the acceptable limits of scholarly rigour and genuine illumination does such talk of virtue and goodness take us? To look for compassion in the coup de grace of the! Kung San, and find it.[7] To look for ambitious hope in the production lines of Foxconn, and find it.[8] To seek courage in the eyes of dogs and find an overflowing source.[9] Perhaps not so far; not when these virtues are taken as instances of something quite general in character, something vitally constitutive of our way of talking about goodness. Just reasonable suspicions.

With this sort of virtue in mind, it may well seem most sensible to take as our models of well-lived lives, those who dedicate themselves most explicitly to the service of others. Charity workers, battlefield nurses, saints in the far-flung hells of humanity; but this will not be the case. To take such lives as exemplars supposes that those sorts of activities are indeed the most virtuous and whilst it shan't be claimed that they are not, establishing their status at this stage would require a tangential discussion of supererogation.[10] Taking perfection as a point of reference creates an awkward need to draw clear boundaries around any possible fault, to tidy up all the cracks, and (as will be explored later) goodness (a life lived well) might not only allow for faults but necessarily entail them.

Perhaps, though, the potential for these kinds of shiny lives, and the virtues they demonstrate, to act as sources of inspiration might permit us to draw a common thread between the virtues they express. 'Selflessness' might be the title of that theme. Certainly, the problems of where to stop, of the importance of self-regard, of the place of non-sentient entities; these all worm their way into any theory of selflessness as a fulcrum of ethics. But perhaps a concept like 'selflessness', however grand, vague and problematic, could be sufficiently solid so as to serve, at least in the first instance, as 'the criterion by which we judge the reasonableness of our suspicion that a life is being lived properly or well'.

Perhaps it is the nature of reasonable suspicion when it is playing an important guiding role in an investigation which involves practical as well as conceptual enquiry, that much of its more nuanced and detailed character (as much as it may ever be detailed) emerges through practice. As will be seen below (and particularly in relation to the work of Albert Schweitzer) selflessness brings its own important conflicts and it is just these sorts of conflicts (conceptual, practical and ethical) which can act as the greatest lessons in wisdom (virtue and wellbeing).

Experts in living and thinking

So far, then, this discussion might be summarised (in a perhaps less than generous fashion) thus:

1   There is a virtue, 'wisdom', which is the traditional and best goal of philosophy and which some people possess more than others, some aspect of this virtue is (to at least some extent) within reach of all of us (at least humans) and it can be increased.

2 Wisdom both entails and is fostered by living a better more moral life and by seeking a greater understanding of how to do this.

3 Wisdom has something to do with a broad and enquiring perspective on the world and on those with whom one shares it.

4 To increase wisdom, it is necessary to gain this greater perspective through a combination of both abstract enquiry and lived experience which must often deal with central and abiding conflicts (to be expanded upon later).

5 This current discussion will conduct this combination of abstract enquiry and lived experience with a particular way of life deemed an apt source of insight.

So general a collection of statements as this could imply an investigation of almost any sort. Doesn't everyone employ this combination of abstraction and direct experience anyway?[11] Such an enquiry would be tantamount to merely creating a written record of human life in its most mundane and general of forms; a stream of consciousness with a vaguely interrogative bent. This brings me to Tim Ingold and his suggestion that anthropology (and a certain kind of philosophy) is just an extension of what everyone does normally anyway. I agree, it is, and so is philosophy, in fact, when done properly, anthropology and philosophy are the same things. This amalgam of philosophy and anthropology will be the means by which this investigation of wisdom and wellbeing will be conducted.

In his article *That's Enough About Ethnography*, Ingold (2014, pp. 383–395) seeks to distinguish what he identifies as the rigid and academically restricted practice of ethnography from the more open-ended and expansive discipline of anthropology or 'participant observation'. Ingold's primary reason for wishing to do this is that he observes a kind of objectification in ethnography which he views as necessarily foreign to participant observation which requires a *'living with'* as opposed to a 'writing about'. Ingold believes that this crucial distinction is frequently forgotten, to the detriment of anthropology. What I agree with here is Ingold's description of participant observation as differing 'only in degree from what all people do all of the time, though children more than most'. I also agree with Ingold that the strength of participant observation is in its openness to difference and cooperative approach to understanding other ways of life. What I disagree with is his suggestion that the sort of 'distortion that contrives to render the aftermath of our meetings with people as their anterior condition', which he identifies with ethnography, is neither a part of participant observation nor (by extension) philosophy and our lives more generally.

Ingold is clear about the continuity and even identity he acknowledges between anthropology and a certain kind of philosophy. Towards the close of his discussion of ethnography, he quotes his own words: 'anthropology is philosophy with the people in' (*Ibid.*, p. 393) I shan't seek to dispute the particular incarnation of philosophy he intends to embrace here, it is enough for now just to find support for the general notion of philosophy as anthropology (and vice versa). What is crucial here is that philosophy is more commonly associated with the sort of distant reflection which Ingold views as detrimental to the process of 'living with' which is the great strength of anthropological investigation (*Ibid.,* p. 389).

What is this practice which is different 'only in degree from what all people do all of the time, though children more than most'? Does such a suggestion entail an overly romanticised view of children? Perhaps some pictures of an innocent face, staring in wide-eyed wonder at the world. Or maybe a little voice asking why the sky is blue, why one rule applies to them and not to another, why the pigs live outside and the dogs inside, why grandma isn't coming back, why we sleep at night and not in the day why, why, why, why, why. Surely, though, we can put this sort of wonder and ceaseless query down to naivety and lack of experience, and we certainly wouldn't want to reduce anthropology or philosophy to a professional infantilism.

The connection between philosophical thinking and a kind of childlike wonder and tendency to question things which are otherwise taken for granted by the stagnant, grown-up masses is not original to Ingold. In the *Theaetetus* Socrates describes how 'wonder is the only beginning of philosophy' (Plato, *Theatetus*, §155d) and Aristotle echoes Plato's thoughts in his Metaphysics when he explains that 'it is because of wonder that men both now begin and first began to philosophise' (Aristotle, *Metaphysics*, §I: II; 982b).[12] Of course, wonder is not the sole preserve of children but we can perhaps see why Ingold would relate the exaggerated form in which it does occur in the young to the practice of participant observation. The wonder of children is born out of freshness, unfamiliarity with their surroundings; anthropologists often seek to place themselves in similarly unfamiliar situations, into environments which they hope will teach them something new.

It is the curious, seemingly contradictory mixture of participation and observation which acts as the focus of Ingold's paper and which is the key to the methodological coextension of philosophy and a social science which this current discussion seeks to establish. Indeed, it will be suggested that this social scientific methodology embodies the very balance of contradiction and coherence which has hitherto been identified with a correct epistemic and ethical attitude. To participate fully in an activity and to simultaneously maintain a reflective disposition which involves considering one's situation from an external perspective is the remit of philosophy.

That the realities of a form of life, social facts, are understood from within has, typically, driven those considering social research to place an emphasis very much on the participation part as opposed to the observation part of this practice. J. H. Gill suggests that Peter Winch's (1958) *The Idea of a Social Science and its Relation to Philosophy* should have been called 'The Very Idea of a Social *Science!*' (Gill 1982, p. 417). Science is one thing, it deals with facts, objective matters, social realities are something quite different. So if we are to understand someone else's perspective, their way of life, we must live that life too, we must participate but we shouldn't hope for any kind of objective observations as part of this participation. Ingold echoes Winch's thoughts in his effort to distance anthropology from ethnography. Objectivity requires an outside perspective, an observation, and we are always on the inside.

J. H. Gill is quite right to wonder why anyone would preserve a special place for the physical sciences (*Ibid., p. 420*). Gill may be right that this is because many thinkers prior to more recent scholarship in the philosophy of mind, failed to consider the enveloping nature of our complex, tangible realities. If we are not rational and physical, but rather ratio-physical, there is continuity between us and the physical world, its rules and our minds are not distinct. Sadly, Gill takes this neglect of our 'embodied' nature to be an excuse to ride the participation wagon all the way into town; no more room for observation. Similarly, Ingold follows this relativistic epistemology to clothe participant observation in the many hues of Heraclytean flux. It is not necessary to travel too far down this epistemic path, that piece has already been said. Instead of reproducing arguments, a case can be made for the kind of strange balance between objectivity and subjectivity, uncertainty and confidence (which has been outlined above) as being far more in line with the super-childlike wonder which Ingold invokes, than the maelstrom of life and perspectives which would result from dissolution of observation.

The insider-outsider distinction (or, indeed, 'problem') has been at the core of many debates in social science.[13] This is the banner under which the dilemma of the 'conversation stopper' mentioned earlier has been academically legitimised. The parent saying 'you can't possibly understand this unless you are a parent' threatens to become the guardian of an insuperable epistemic fortress. This is frequently distilled most potently in the study of religion, where the Elyeusian mysteries of faith do become the sole preserve of the initiate, invulnerable to outside investigation.[14] What the wonder of children can illustrate here is not only an attitude and mental state which is exaggerated and honed in the philosopher-anthropologist but also a position of insider-outsider which illustrates the fallacy of raising any impermeable epistemic membrane.

We might think that, of necessity, there must be a point at which the parent becomes a parent. To assign this process a single 'point', however, is to be overly atomistic. My own becoming a father occurred, and occurs still, in contiguous stages. Prior to the birth of my daughter, the pregnancy was itself composed of these stages, of a growing sense of her imminent arrival, of my wife's shifting sizes and sufferings and, importantly, of the persistent reminder from friends who had children that 'it will change everything'. 'Think you are tired now?... You have no idea'. Really? 'no idea'? 'change everything'? Being of a pedantic and critical disposition these proclamations of epistemic and experiential alterations beyond my possible current understanding raised concerns. Certainly, experiences come in varying magnitudes of significance, changing us more or less, but these, it had seemed to me, are differences in *degree*, not (at least not altogether) in *kind*. During my limited time on earth so far I had never experienced the kind of transformation of which these people spoke, certainly, I had experienced major changes, 'life altering' even, but not a metamorphosis totally without prelude or suggestion. Perhaps this way of speaking is just idiomatic, perhaps they just meant that the change is significant, but I suspect that its proclamation was connected with a sense of pride in knowledge which comes with an idea of removal from the uninitiated. Tribes of knowledge, clubs of experience.

Of course, it wasn't entirely accurate (and perhaps I take too much glee in the affirmation of my own contrary epistemic removal from that folk knowledge). Our daughter's arrival was wonderful, profound, exhausting and terrifying, certainly, but (in part) similar to other things. Before her birth, I had suspected that those who spoke so certainly of the imminent transformation were those with limited experience of looking after other animals or elderly relatives. Those experiences also bring much of the responsibility, emotional turmoil and sleeplessness that parenthood brings. Our daughter has pushed our understanding of these domestic ways of living and thinking to new heights and given us a keen sense of our continuous state of discovery, but that might as well remind us of past discoveries as prompt us to wonder at future ones.

Meno queries how we can possibly discover the answer to a question if we do not already know it, because how will we know where to look and how will we know when we get there? (Plato, *Meno*, §80d-e) It is an epistemic variation of Zeno's paradox, where Achilles must traverse an infinite number of points before he can reach his goal. If any journey is composed of increments, and those increments are similarly composed of increments, and so on, then an impenetrable barrier is established to any kind of progression. If our discoveries are preceded by other related discoveries then how do we move from one to the next? What drives us from ignorance to knowledge? Must we simply be passive receptors of experience? Motes without agency drifting through a cloud of life?

The problem is to imagine any dynamic system (physical or otherwise) as of necessity being composed of atoms or points. We can recognise distinct things, bodies and events, in the universe and this leads us to imagine that the universe is composed entirely of distinct things and this leaves the relationships between those distinct things as a vexatious, infinitely regressive problem. Instead, let us imagine discovery as a matter of betweenness. What is meant here is largely an application of a kind of process philosophy.[15] To reject Epicurean atomism of the universe is frequently imagined to be synonymous with adopting either a Parmenidean mysticism whereby identity and form is some kind of epiphenomenal trick of psychology or a Heraclytean dedication to chaos whereby identity and form are similarly consigned to illusion. Process ontology is usually associated with the latter view but allows for identities to emerge from the chaos, and this is just the compromise necessary to make sense of the activity of learning, to merge participation and observation. To cultivate wonder (or resurrect it) is not to abandon oneself to a state of boundless drift but to float with direction, to navigate with rudder, sail and anchor.

We are, each of us, always in a process between knowledge and ignorance, a half-way-house of constantly dawning realisation. The horizon of understanding shifts as we shift, some of its epistemic landmarks are more dramatic than others but mountains of the mind don't just rise up out of nowhere, their shining peaks appear long before we glimpse their vast and complex roots. We needn't commit to the meaningless dreamscape (or nightmare) of total experiential flux, nor the Platonic solidity of predetermined knowledge. We can have both; things that change, *relatedness and difference*.

And, of course, it must be so; children show us this. Wonder and ceaseless interrogation are the visible and audible manifestation of this state of constant discovery. Things are new but they are also identifiable, phenomena fit into increasingly definite frameworks of meaning, language games are played more and more adeptly. If this learning occurred either solely through the passive reception of novel revelations or through pure extrapolation from familiar perspectives then no wonder would be extant. What impact could any realisation have if it were utterly distinct from a child's previous understanding if it didn't *fit*? As William James says:

> The novelty soaks in; it stains the ancient mass; but it is also tinged by what absorbs it. Our past apperceives and co-operates; and in the new equilibrium in which each step forward in the process of learning terminates, it happens relatively seldom that the new fact is added *raw*. More usually it is embedded cooked, as one might say, or stewed down in the sauce of the old.
>
> (James 1907, p. 78)

I might write or speak, ehnghsplit, a sentence which has a hitherto unknown word in it and those witness to this novelty won't experience wonder, merely confusion (and possibly irritation). Similarly, if one moment to the next were only populated by the drawing out of previous moments then no change would ever really occur. Wonder is the spirit of adventure, not of sheer novelty. The pure invention has a disjointed and monstrous quality to it, again it smells like the hubris and bloated pride of one who views creation itself as the most divine of acts rather than the humility of learning.

But a pattern is observed, from novelty to familiarity. Fresh-faced youth subsides into the world-weary, safe mediocrity of age. To this the philosopher objects, she objects because it is dishonest. To treat any knowledge as complete would be to deny its relatedness to that which is unknown, to project it as an atom of understanding. What the anthropologist does, what the philosopher does, is refuse to allow this process of discovery to ossify, to reject that safety of a single way of seeing things and instead, look around the corner of the world for a new view. We are inexorably drawn into our own way of seeing the world and the outsiderishness of childhood is worn away by the distractions of familiarity.

Let's extend the landscape metaphor.[16]

Perhaps this deterioration of wonder happens because the peaks of the mountaintops are just so brilliant and majestic, the dark and tangled roots at their feet are barely even visible to those who have looked skyward for so long. If we take our time, though, and acclimatise to the detail of that which lies beneath the highlights of our world, if we peer through the misty darkness of the forests and valleys, we will find endlessly branching valleys and streams, waterways which spread far and wide and which, ultimately, intertwine with new, previously unguessed-at sources and pinnacles, distant caps which invite us to continue our journey with renewed vigour.

What the anthropologist-philosopher must *not* do is consider herself a pure participant and forget that the new mountain is linked to the last by the valleys below. Ways of living and thinking isolated from one another by a void and into which one must simply throw oneself. Ingold is in danger of suggesting it is all peaks; the analysis, the 'anterior condition', what lies beneath the snow and sun, these are the means by which we reach the next discovery, flying from peak to peak, blown by the wind any which way, that is as much a problem as the analyst, the detached philosopher, the ethnographer, who reduces the mountain to its geology, the worldview to its justifications and causes, who spends their life digging to the very core of the earth only to be burned to nothing in the process or who merely digs in their 'work time' and treats their mine as imaginary, or ancillary upon emerging. The fruitful path, the holistic, big-picture approach is one of stone *and* sky.

Certainly we may need to push ourselves sometimes, to jump from a secure place towards a new way of life, and we might only get a proper look at the foundations in their entirety when we are actually squarely atop that new rise, but we mustn't forget what lies below.

Which is to say:

1 There is a manner in which seemingly isolated world views are connected through their foundations.
  A These foundations are the justifications, rationales, moral observations, psychological tendencies, biological and environmental universals upon which (and of which) our knowledge is built.
2 Philosophical analysis has traditionally taken as its objects of interest these unseen foundations.
3 The process of engaging in that sort of analysis requires removal from the well-defined comfort and familiarity of the assumptions and well-established knowledge of a particular perspective or way of life.
4 This removal, this observation, must usually be orchestrated if it is to be manifested beyond an intuitive and immediate unfamiliarity with the world (that sort demonstrated by children).

5 This orchestration of observation must be tethered to participation, and the participation to an observation if it is to achieve the broad, holistic knowledge which it traditionally and properly sets as its goal and this is what is meant by an exaggeration of 'what all people do all of the time, though children more than most.'[17]

This does have practical implications. This discussion of participant observation has been framed as a criticism of Tim Ingold but in truth, that opposition is somewhat artificial. Ingold's real objection to ethnography is the way in which it is taught as some kind of special activity, almost a scientific experiment which is prepared, conducted and completed (with conclusions flowing thenceforth) (Ingold 2014, p. 387). Prior to the ethnographic research, one is not doing ethnography and afterwards one can resume one's 'normal', non-anthropological life. Ingold rejects this view of anthropology and sets out the way in which there cannot be a strict division between fieldwork and non-fieldwork (*Ibid.*, p. 386). The similarities between this objection and the efforts of philosophy as a way of life are not, I w ould suggest, coincidental and one key purpose of this current chapter is to establish why and how these two seemingly distant academic schools of thought are, in fact, of one mind.

Both are rejections of the professionalism and specialism which has come to dominate and define the academy. The view that there is a core, universal principle of learning and self-improvement through a greater understanding of the world and, crucially, those with whom we share it, is at the heart of both disciplines and, one might argue (indeed philosophy as a way of life does so argue), at the heart of the academy itself (or at least historically so). The academic enquiry becomes, by the standards of these anti-specialist schools of thought, a kind of refinement of human conduct, a distillation of being a reflexive being. Instead of a pastime, it is an ethos which bleeds into all aspects of life.

The claim then, on the face of it, is a simple one. The dichotomy between practical and theoretical knowledge is a false one. Just as with the rejection of the dichotomy between knowledge and doubt; however, this rejection must itself be mitigated, it might even be said that the dichotomy between dichotomy and unity is itself a false dichotomy. Once again the perennial dilemma of philosophy, of bipolarity, rears its head; the inescapable shadows of Heraclitus and Parmenides.

It would be foolish and self-refuting, however, to at once repudiate the over-intellectualisation of philosophical investigation and simultaneously declaim the necessary conjunction of intellectual abstraction and practical engagement. Instead, perhaps, another metaphor (poles can do the job of dichotomies): A sphere has poles, antipodes, yet from its innermost core to its broadest surface, these opposing points are conjoined. Indeed, the very idea of an object *as such* involves this concurrence of opposed points and unified conjunction and so too might this ontological precondition be extended to epistemic states. Distant and careful reflection, abstraction, rigorous cogitation, these things can and do occur in stark and seemingly isolated contrast from the almost unthinking, automatic, visceral, sensuous absorption of the world and its activities; but *'almost'* is the key term here. Even on those occasions when these ways of learning are most distant from one another, they are not detached, for if they were, they would cease to have a definition, just as if one side of a coin were to vanish so too, of necessity, would the other.

What is being claimed is not the impossibility of abstract reflection, of part-time conceptual analysis, or purely descriptive, professional social science. Such a denial of what is quite obviously extant would be odd at best; preposterous would probably be nearer the mark. The claim here is primarily normative, not empirical, it is that when the goal of one's investigation is something very broad, perhaps the broadest of all possible goals, that of 'life, the universe and everything', as Douglas Adams might put it (Adams 1982) then the best approach is one which deals not in epistemic extremes, niches, specialties or parts but, rather, in *wholes*. The goal of this book, of achieving a better understanding of wisdom and wellbeing, is indeed a goal of just this sort of breadth. If wisdom is understood as an understanding (a perception and practice) of what is most important, then the sweep of our net must be as wide as we can muster.

By way of objection to this attempted union of philosophical reflection and anthropological methods, it might be suggested that the idea of self-cultivation, self-improvement even, is not by any means an integral aspect of social scientific enquiry and that it is with this principle that the similarity between these two movements ends. Furthermore, if the kind of realism which has been suggested as integral (or at least very helpful) to the ancient model of wisdom is indeed accepted as part of the philosophical way of life then the two traditions might be seen as thrust even further apart. Any such objection would, however, in order that it might be accurate, require an opponent seeking union in history rather than potential. What I mean here is that (as with the previous analysis of Aristotle and Plato) my intent is normative rather than exegetical. It is what is common between these emerging traditions which interests me, as it is that which I wish to put forward as fruitful. Just as with Plato and Aristotle, it is principally in their points of convergence that I am suggesting greatest wisdom can be gleaned.

If, however, one were inclined to humour such an objection, there are good reasons to reject this idea that evaluation and moral judgment are not common to both philosophy and participant observation. Even in a purely descriptive sense, what is discovered, what is sought in any process of mindfully living with others, is a cohesive 'way of life': a tune to which people dance. One cannot truly participate, live life amongst others, without learning their language game and their 'form of life'. Wittgenstein certainly recognised how close he was bringing philosophy to social science yet still he wished to maintain a division based on reflective distance. He explains:

If we look at things from an ethnological point of view, does that mean we are saying philosophy is ethnology? No, it only means that we are taking up a position right outside so as to be able to see things more objectively.

(Wittgenstein 1940, p. 37)

Wittgenstein is commenting here on the sort of comparative 'ethnology' found in Frazer's (1890) *Golden Bough*, rather than the reflections of participant observation, and perhaps this is partly to blame for his adversarial tone.[18] Yet Wittgenstein's desire to retain distance is linked to an insistence that a form of life must be considered as a cohesive whole if it is to be understood at all. As Antonio Marques remarks, Wittgenstein sought 'the peculiar connections of a whole form of life' (Marques 2010, p. 64).

Now, it may seem quite a leap to move from this cohesion of distinct life forms to the insistence that the method for investigating lifeforms must be evaluative. Indeed, it might fairly be thought that some trickery is being attempted in drawing out an ought from an is. By reflecting on a way of life we may well be able to say that this *is* how things are done by these people or those people, but surely we cannot so easily drift into saying that *therefore* this is how things *should* be done.

In the following chapter it will be suggested that there is a continuum between the cohesion of a way of life and moral and aesthetic cohesion and that understanding such cohesion is key to all understanding, moral and otherwise. The culmination of both the epistemology and methodology described thus far will need to be something which ties together these otherwise disparate ways of making sense of things.

When we come to cultivate participant observation (rather than practice it) we are learning to have conversations, to work together, to negotiate impasses of understanding and interests. I am not attempting to suggest that there is anything as monolithic and solid as 'a culture' or a uniform or homogenous way of life which is devoid of inconsistencies, variation and change, quite the reverse. It is precisely these sorts of inconsistencies which make the business of participant-observation-philosophy (what I will call 'living-with') so integral to all life. What I am suggesting is that the negotiation of these cracks in the cohesion of our lives is only possible if one allows for a sort of sensitivity to cohesion as such: practical, psychological, moral and conceptual.[19]

Notes

1 w is necessarily some U but w is some W Iff it is I but since W is I it seems reasonable to suggest that w is I. That this raises the problem of Russell's paradox is hardly a problem at this point (seeing as though paradoxes are already being embraced quite openly, if moderately). On Russell's paradox (and its history and relationship with other paradoxes) see Griffin's (2004, pp. 349–372) *The Prehistory of Russell's Paradox*.

2 On infanticide amongst the Ayoreo see P. E. Bugos and McCarthy's (1984, pp. 504–511) *Ayoreo Infanticide: A Case Study.*

3 Unlike Nicholas White, I do think that the theory of recollection has the potential to form the basis of this moderation (or 'solution') (White 1994, p. 163). I should hasten to add that the form which this theory would take would not the be the theological one which Plato expresses but, rather, a psychological/anthropological/narrative kind of the sort expressed later in this discussion. There is a kind of recollection in the way we recognise coherence, that which we observe fits that which have already at our disposal. (See Plato, *Meno*, pp. 35–72).

4 It will be noted that life being 'done properly' and 'lived well' are two phrases being used synonymously here.

5 For translation, the 'Revised Oxford' entry by Jowett (1995) was consulted.

6 'Virtue in the principal sense' or 'general goodness'.

7 On the ethos of !Kung San hunting see Hurn's (2012, p. 58) *Humans and Other Animals.*

8 I certainly do not mean, here, to undermine in any way the appalling working conditions which many Foxconn employees find themselves subjected to. I would not wish to suggest that these conditions in some way foster the cultivation of particular virtues. The point, rather, is that without reflecting on justice, but also hope and ambition and the full gamut of ethics, little sense can be made of the humans who live and work in Foxconn's factories. Not only is ethics appropriate in these investigations, but it is also necessary. On the lives of those working for organisations like Foxconn, see Ngai's (2016, pp. 181–184) *Incomplete Subjects: Circular Migration and the Life and Death Struggles of the Migrant Workers in China.*

9 The issue of non-human virtue is integral to this book as a whole and will be expanded upon below. In this regard (and others) the work of Raimond Gaita (2003) in *The Philosopher's Dog* has been invaluable. Gaita's reflections on his dog Gypsy offer an example of just this kind of discussion of non-human virtue and it may be worth noting at this point that Gaita remarks explicitly that Gypsy, though she may have been 'An intelligent dog, is not a wise one' (p. 43).

10 I think it is important to note here a line of thought which suggests that charitable giving does not require (or legitimately suggest) supererogation and that the kind of thinking which is appropriate about charity is not anything based on exceptional heroism but, rather, something more calculated and focused on the collective. Toby Ord is, I think, of particular importance in this regard in his 'Giving What we Can' project aims at fostering this kind of group-thinking (Ord, 2008).

11 Always allowing for differences of capacity ([dis]ability is one concern here, species is another, both shall be discussed below).

12 Aristotle, *Metaphysics,* H. Tredennick (tr.), (Cambridge, MA, Harvard University Press, 1933).

13 Clifford Geertz' (1974, pp. 26–45) essay on this topic *'From the Native's Point of View': On the Nature of Anthropological Understanding* is a seminal expression of this enveloping discussion. In its own small way, this current discussion seeks to identify philosophy as a way of life within this same debate about insider vs. outsider.

14 On this impermeability in the study of religion see R. T. McCutcheon's (2005, pp. 67–73) *The Autonomy of Religious Experience.*

15 This needs to be understood in a fairly weak sense. Metaphysical theory, whilst not being discounted as potentially insightful and ultimately necessary, is not something which this discussion can pursue to any great extent. The lack of detailed analysis here of process metaphysics and the philosophy of

Alfred North Whitehead (1929) is similar to the neglect elsewhere of theories of embodied cognition. An attempt is being made, neither to expound any kind of original metaphysics nor a comprehensive analysis of a metaphysical theory, but to supply sufficient cursory mention of those metaphysical topics which pertain more directly to the ethical discussion as to make that ethics less jarring for those who naturally desire some metaphysical basis. The concern here is largely epistemological and psychological. Given the Platonic, (or Murdochian) and Schweitzerian tones of this book, I have no doubt that complimentary metaphysical theory could yield some insight but this would be a task for a library of later treatments, not this one small discussion. I agree with Whitehead (1929, §1:1:1) that a complete philosophy is the desired goal and that such a 'speculative philosophy' should attempt to supply us with something in light of which 'every element of our experience can be interpreted'. On the degree to which Whitehead's philosophy itself contains ethics, see: J. W. Lango's (2001, pp. 515–536) wonderfully entitled *Does Whitehead's Metaphysics Contain an Ethics?*.

16 The extensive use of metaphors, images and poetic language will be excused later.

17 T. Ingold (2014), *That's Enough About Ethnography*, p. 387.

18 Though one might think his reaction would be more violent towards a method involving far more emersion.

19 It may well now be appropriate to recognise the degree to which this talk of cohesion (based as it is in the idea of transcendent boundaries to our existence) resembles some fairly 'old fashioned' forms of phenomenology. Kant's project and later (and far more obviously related) Hegel's *Phenomenology of Spirit* certainly ask many of the same questions and offer similar answers (Hegel 1807). I hope that this is no surprise since one of the central tenets of this book (and hardly a novel suggestion) is that philosophy deals with perennial problems and should aim not for creative originality in the usual sense but rather continuous moral learning through somewhat novel approaches to ancient problems. A future extension of this discussion would undoubtedly call for a more extensive treatment of these early phenomenologies but for now, such exegesis is narrowly beyond the remit of this book.

5 The necessity of aesthetics and evaluation, and the pre-eminence of narrative in 'living-with'

Could beauty, my lord, have better commerce than with honesty?

(Shakespeare, *Hamlet*, 3.1)

μονώτης εἰμί φιλομυθότερος γέγονα.

(Aristotle, from Demetrius' *De Elocutione*[1])

διὸ καὶ ὁ φιλόμυθος φιλόσοφός πώς ἐστιν: ὁ γὰρ μῦθος σύγκειται ἐκ θαυμασίων.

(Aristotle, *Metaphysics*, §1, 982b[2])

It is important to emphasise at the outset of this chapter that the efforts at methodological consilience which are being made in this book are not exclusive in their prescription. This is only to repeat that I do not wish to claim that philosophy *cannot* be something different from anthropology (the word might be used in another way), only that it *can* be the same thing and that when it is it is valuable. My wish is to find common elements which point towards a particularly holistic kind of investigation into a particularly holistic kind of subject. Certainly, definition, finitude, clear and practical limitations are not only a useful part of interrogatory methods but a necessary part of all meaningful concepts. My suggestion (though it is not really my own for it is a staple of the history of philosophy) is that a definitive and central aspect of philosophy is to attempt to deal with the most general and expansive concepts it can manage. As the primary focus of this book, I have taken one of the most general concepts (wisdom) and understood this itself to be defined by what may be *the most* general of concepts ('The Good').[3] I have taken as compelling to the point of being axiomatic Aristotle's suggestion that a method of investigation should mirror its subject matter and desired goals in both detail and breadth. As such, I have attempted to outline, with an appropriate degree of perspicuity, an understanding of philosophy whereby this discipline is itself best suited in means to its proclaimed ends.

In as far as this investigation has attempted to reflect the generality and multifarious nature of its subject it may have been so far suspected of being occasionally unnecessarily opaque, diffuse and even verbose in its means and expression. This chapter, in attempting to tie together the methodological, metaethical and epistemological section of this book, will also attempt to address these concerns of style and substance. This will serve as the fourth and final point of the propaedeutic to part two of this book in which the investigation proper into wisdom and permaculture will take place.

Rhetoric! This is the word most likely to be thrown at any effort to persuade which does not follow those means and modes of argument traditionally adhered to by modern (we might even say 'analytic') philosophy. The charge here is likely to be one of evasion and dishonesty, a betrayal of the core principles of philosophy. Rhetoric is concerned with persuasion, not truth; rhetoric concerns itself with the relationship between the point being put across and the audience, not with the *justifications* for this point. If there were a cheap trick to ensure an audience's conversion, rhetoric would use it.[4]

In what follows I am happy to indulge this somewhat two-dimensional view of rhetoric, I am even happy to conflate rhetoric with sophistry as this view seems bound to do. The reason for this easy indulgence is that the theory that there is an inappropriate and anti-philosophical (dishonest) way to attempt persuasion and even engage in interrogation is useful to this current discussion. For the time being, it really doesn't matter what we call this anti-philosophy, this charm masquerading as wisdom, what matters is the 'true philosophy' against which it is measured.

'Poetry' is one term that might be used to describe something else besides rhetoric, 'song' is another, 'stories' and 'storytelling' are yet other possible terms for the same sort of thing, 'myth' and 'mythopoesis' are others still. These are the terms which best capture the central topic of this chapter and part of its efforts will be in distinguishing this 'storytelling' from that less scrupulous form of philosophy which might be identified with rhetoric or sophistry. In what follows, some of these terms will be used somewhat interchangeably. Certainly, 'poetry', 'myth' and 'story' all have different connotations, but what they have in common is that which is most crucial. The different connotations will be put to use and each term will be employed in slightly different contexts though it is important to note that these differences are far less important than that which is common. As a working definition it will be useful to make use of Robert Burch's attempt to clarify the difference between philosophy and poetry:

> Suffice it to remind ourselves that, since Nietzsche and Heidegger, no one can simply take for granted the divisions and determinations of the apophantic and aesthetic upon which this usual definition of the poetic turns, nor the ready equation of poetry with meter and verse that it posits. Instead, to begin with, we understand the term 'poetic' here in the broadest etymological sense to encompass the whole domain of *poesis*

as that of the creative production of meaning. Following etymology, we likewise construe the term 'philosophy' in a similarly broad way as *philosophia*, the love of wisdom, expressed in the quest for *truth*.

(Burch 2002, p. 3)

Here, less emphasis will be placed on the 'creative production' element of ποίησις (at least in the sense of the autonomous or purposeful act of a person) and far more on the sense of the emergence (purposeful or otherwise) of meaning and the contiguous nature of this emergence. As has already been explained, the understanding of philosophy here links the quest for truth inseparably to a quest for improvement through an increase in one's ability to recognise significance (chiefly moral) and act accordingly. It is through these ideas of significance and meaning that a union of poetry and philosophy will be described.

At the centre of this discussion of poetry (and particularly what we might call stories or myth) is an attempt to tie together both the means of investigation and argument exercised in this book and the kind of growth in (cultivation of) wisdom through living-with as discussed in the previous chapter. It will be argued that just as participant observation grants us windows into truth, and rigorous and logical argument and investigation also grants us a view of truth, so too can beauty offer similar revelation. It will be suggested that it is here that a general species of cohesion, a 'hanging-together', can be identified, that it this which characterises all of these modes of understanding and that it is, for this reason, they (should) all share a persuasiveness. Aesthetic awareness is the third part to 'living-with'.

A conflict to resolve

Our history must always begin with a battle.

It is an age of heroes, of wine-dark seas, and the coast of Asia Minor (as ever it seems to be) is alive with the clamour of a human tempest. Bronze flashes, empires rise and fall. Here identities are born. One history begins with gods fighting men, another with men fighting gods.

Apollo, 'arrows rattling on the shoulders of the angry god as he moves', unleashes merciless death amongst the Greek host (Homer, *Iliad*, §1:45). Sometime later (and 177 miles further south) Thales wonders if things might not, in fact, be somewhat different from the way the poets have hitherto suggested. With less spectacle and glamour Thales unleashes far more devastating arrows. Unlike Achilles, Thales is not supported by a mighty army, his Myrmidons were yet to come. One of them, Socrates, greatest of their number, appears armed for the same cause, standing against the monstrous name of custom, against a tide of comfort and fear, he aims blows against deception and perishes in the effort, yet his battle cries echoed on and shaped a world entire.

If any clear view of philosophy as myth is to be achieved then we must first overcome the immediate objection that philosophy, by definition, was the opposite of myth, and that's how it was born and continues to function.[5] For a better understanding of this history, that philosophy arose in explicit opposition to religious and poetic tradition, we must again turn to Aristotle and Plato. At the outset of the *Metaphysics*, as Aristotle is attempting to outline the nature of his subject matter (the nature of wisdom and philosophy), he turns to a brief history of philosophy and to Thales and (notably) Hesiod at its inception. He describes how the first philosophers were all concerned with finding a single principle at the source of all things and that Thales identified this principle with water:

> There are some who think the men of very ancient times, long before the present era, who first speculated about the gods, also held this same opinion about the primary entity. For they represented Oceanus and Tethys to be the parents of creation... they say that this was Thales' opinion concerning the first cause.
>
> (Aristotle, *Metaphysics*, §I: III; 983b1–984a5)

After considering the shortfalls of theories which place a material element as the first principle, Aristotle goes on to say that philosophers now needed to ask what kind of non-material principle might be at the root of things and that:

> It might be inferred that the first person to consider this question was Hesiod... for Hesiod says –
> First of all things was Chaos made, and then
> Broad bosomed Earth...
> And Love, the foremost of immortal beings
> Thus implying that there must be in the world some cause to move things and combine them.
>
> (*Ibid.*, §I: IV; 984b23–31)[6]

Two things are important to draw from these accounts (and also that which serves as the second epigraph to this chapter in which Aristotle draws a similarity between myth, loving and philosophy): (1) That poetry/storytelling and religion are, in this context, synonymous (this is why the word 'myth' will be of some, albeit limited, use) and (2) Both philosophy and myth are concerned with the same questions (principally, in their infancy, the structure and content of the cosmos: physics and metaphysics, the wisdom of Apollo). Both of these (related) points will be of some consequence for this discussion of wisdom. The first point will, at this juncture, only be significant as a point of information and clarification. When speaking of poetry and storytelling in an ancient Greek context what we are talking about is a

Pre-Socratic tradition intimately bound up with the metaphysical, ethical and historical beliefs of the Hellenes, not an idle or merely aesthetic practice. The second point is of more immediate concern. The idea that philosophy is opposed to myth is rooted in an idea of the two arts as vying over the same territory and that their mastery of that ground is mutually exclusive; it is this mutual exclusivity which I wish, in part, to dispute.[7] It is this conflict which is most clearly articulated by Plato's discussion of the 'ancient quarrel between philosophy and poetry' (Plato, *Republic*, 607b5–6)[8] and which is at the root of the case he puts forward for philosophy against poetry and rhetoric.

The territory under dispute is that of the immaterial, the powerful, the important, *The Truth*. This is the stuff of wisdom: important things. The poets had been the formulators and disseminators of the truth amongst the Hellenes for time immemorial and though it was inventive and adaptive in the sense of speaking to the people and reflecting their own world, it was static in its means and pompous in its claims to authority. Philosophy was a rebellion against the status quo of received authority. Perhaps, rather than just regurgitating old stories, they thought, we could augment these stories with inquiry and observation (I think 'augment' is the right word here, as will be seen). As Barfield suggests, it was discontent with mere particulars which drove this rebellion (Barfield 2011, p. 12). It's all well and good if the gods bind their vows by the water of The Styx, but what is the water doing? How does it do it? Is it at the foundation of other things? *All* things? These lovers of wisdom sought not the isolated fragments of the cosmos but the wholes which they compose, the points of their origin and the lines along which they run.

It may be apparent in this account of myth and philosophy that though I am attempting to move away from a view of opposition I am not trying to dissolve conflict. 'Rebellion' may indeed be too strong a word; even by the time of Aristotle, it was evidently still permissible for a philosopher to turn to a poet for insight (however limited that insight might be).

Plato's republic is to be free of poets but they are replaced by philosophers (Plato *Republic*, 377d). Rebellions come in many forms. Certainly, the vitriol of Plato's *Republic* might make us think this rebellion against myth is of the nature of replacement but development might be nearer the mark. We do not think of Einstein as being opposed to Newton, of Galileo as an enemy of Ptolemy. It might, however, be suggested that Einstein and Newton shared a method and goal and only differed in their solutions, we might say something similar to Galileo and Ptolemy. Perhaps this is why we think of philosophy and storytelling as being so opposed, we imagine that *their methods and goals are distinct* and that the conflict must be one of opposition rather than of development. The development model might just fail to fit.

It is not too hard to see the modern opposition between science and religion as being the successor to the quarrel between philosophy and myth, we might even say it is identical.

As much as this tension between science and religion might be seen as crude and populist it is nonetheless very real.[9] I have, in the past, been tasked with challenging this idea of an inherent conflict between science and religion with school-aged children; it is a less than a simple process. The majority of the children whom I have taught tend to think this battle is a foregone conclusion (though they may sit on differing sides of the divide). My go-to sources for this effort in reconciliation are His Holiness Tenzin Gyatso, the 14th Dalai Lama, and the 104th Archbishop of Canterbury, Rowan Williams. Apart from being two figures for whom I have a great deal of respect and admiration (and whom I, therefore, relish introducing children to at the earliest opportunity) these two figures are also prominent religious leaders who have been outspoken about the natural synergy between religion and science. The reason this is of particular relevance at this juncture is that the kind of synergy which these figures (and others of like-minds) discuss may offer a response to the objection that philosophy and storytelling are at-odds or cannot be brought together.

One possible problem with this model of cooperation between science and religion is that it typically imagines the universe as carved up into different kinds of questions, some of which can be answered by science and others by religion. As Rowan Williams explains:

> It is a complete falsehood to suggest that there is an intrinsic hostility between the scientific worldview and religious faith... Many modern scientists have supposed that when they do their scientific research they are speaking from a position of, you might say, synoptic understanding of how the world works so that the most basic, fundamentally true way of talking about the world is in terms of material interaction. That reductive approach is perhaps the most generative of conflict between scientists and people of faith, at least as the media and popular intellectual communication presents it.
>
> (Williams 2012, p. 3)

It would probably also be fair to say that the sin goes both ways and there are plenty of religious leaders and 'people of faith' who also attempt to be all things to all men. Either someone says all things can be reduced to the material or the other says that all things can be reduced to the immaterial. The crucial concern that this model raises is that we have already seen how philosophy, since its inception, has explicitly concerned itself with being holistic, universal and exhaustive. First-principles are, by their nature, somewhat reductive. So a synergistic model of reconciliation between philosophy and storytelling may also fail since synergy requires sharing and philosophy appears to be a greedy habit.

If the development model of conflict resolution fails and the synergy model also falls short, perhaps this battle is doomed to end in misery. If, however, some accommodation of both models could be made, then perhaps philosophy as storytelling might better survive this introduction.

If philosophy is science *and* poetry then perhaps it can be all things to all men. It can make claims on all topics *because it does so with some circumspection*, to poetry it is science and to science it is poetry. When it finds a poem of gods and magic it introduces statistics, when it finds cold, hard facts it asks after the soul. The idea of synergy is that certain questions are part of one domain, and others of another. Perhaps this can be utilised, not in terms of the subject matter so much as a scale. It is not hard to see how sciences can hive off from philosophy by this means and in this way (historically) also sit comfortably with a developmental model of philosophy. When the question is not 'What is change?' but rather 'What causes *this* change?' we can see a difference in scale, between universal and particular, which renders one philosophy and the other science. This is the difference in the sort of question to which commentators like Rowan Williams wish to draw our attention.

It may be harder to understand, however, how this would work with philosophy and storytelling. Perhaps, in maintaining the non-exclusivity of this argument, we could also allow some non-philosophical storytelling. These would need to be the kind of stories which make no effort in drawing our attention to universals. As will be discussed in the next section, however, this book will again follow Plato, this time in suggesting that such two-dimensional, hollow creations are (at least when they exist, and sadly they frequently do) vicious and the enemy of true philosophy. It is in this sense that the idea of development is most useful, to express the way in which philosophy should be understood as the 'new' poetry. Good stories need to be true stories (though perhaps 'truth stories' would be a better term since these need to be stories which communicate some truth as opposed to stories which, in their entirety, depict events which truly occurred).

Ultimately, when discussing philosophy as storytelling, I am not attempting to peel back the millennia and suggest that it would somehow have been better if the Milesians hadn't bothered; rather, I am attempting to suggest that in setting its escape trajectory too directly away from myth (at least in the analytic tradition), philosophy has lost something which it would do well to reclaim by an at least partial return. The Milesian and more generally classical reaction against the religious authority of the poets was productive of a new critical way of thinking and it is right that we should see science as *an* inheritor of this tradition but just because this movement has been fruitful, its linear continuation need not be so. Philosophy certainly added something to ancient storytelling but it does not follow that it must have erased something. Perhaps anthropology and its storytelling can be seen as an effort to restrain philosophy from destroying itself through this linear movement (this is indeed how I would suggest anthropology should be seen).

Of course, people, *The People*, have always found comfort in traditions and stories which paint pretty pictures, which capture the imagination.

Rhapsodes and their ilk had been peddling smoke and mirrors long before the Sophists ever got their grubby hands on the tools of logical argumentation and critical dialogue. Indeed, it has already been suggested here that the proper place of philosophy is precise to draw people away from the comfort of the familiar, to introduce new ways of thinking, of seeing the world. To imagine, however, that the rejection of received wisdom requires the rejection of all the means and content of that wisdom is to confuse matters; to throw the baby out with the bathwater. It is certainly not terribly novel to suggest that stories, myths even, can reveal uncomfortable, unfamiliar realities. If we are to attempt a return to philosophy as a way of life, a revival of ancient styles of philosophy, then we also need to understand the way in which ancient philosophy can be seen as having built upon myth rather than destroying it. Nor, indeed, does a rejection of comfort, and the authority which exploits comfort, necessarily entail a rejection of all the passions associated with storytelling. We are moved by tales and poetry in many ways, not least by the unveiling of truth, and this passion for truth (if nothing else) is at the very core of philosophy.

Bad art and 'thick-psychology'

It's always a fight and there has always been philosophy. Why should we imagine it was a new thing? Because the Greeks gave it a name? Certainly, a written tradition of philosophy, in Greek, Chinese or Sanskrit emerges at a particular time, but it doesn't follow that before that time nobody thought critically, that nobody sought out goodness and truth and beauty in a careful, compassionate, rigorous and critical manner. That such written traditions have emerged in isolated enclaves of wisdom would suggest that the tendency was at least latent, if not persistent. I see no reason to believe that there have not always been philosophers, though they may have been more or less common and are now nameless and voiceless.[10] They have always been opposed on two sides. Just as with the idea of moderation in conviction with which this discussion began, philosophy has always been hemmed in by the forces of comfort and greed, the collective and the superman, blind devotion and empty selfishness, dogma and nihilism. Tell the people to question their beliefs and you are struck down, tell a king to fight for virtue, not profit, and you are struck down. The temptation may be to imagine a sudden break with traditions of storytelling, poetry, art and myth because these seem timeless and written philosophy so novel. This discussion of wisdom, however, requires a vision of philosophy that permits it to be as timeless as people and their stories because it *is* people and their stories.

Why can't poetry just be art? Pure wordy creation? Sure, poetry might have been a religious myth in ancient Greece and current religion is just a mix of those kinds of myths and some pseudo-philosophy, but why do you need philosophy and myth to be the same thing? Can't stories just be inventions for fun? Entertainment? Can't their cohesion, their hanging together, just be a matter of mere taste and the satisfaction of appetites? Certainly, stories, poetry and (if you really insist) myth can contain truth, but this is just a sugar coating for truths which could be more perspicuously expressed through philosophical argument. That is the whole point of philosophy, it attempts to get away from all the fluff and foggy padding which is found in so much art. The point of those arts, when they do contain truths or moral content (and that is far from necessary) is to be easier for the majority of people to consume, or at least just to offer them variety in their intellectual diet.

It might be entirely plausible to simply dismiss this voice of criticism as yet another incarnation of relativism, of sophistry and rhetoric, those ancient enemies of philosophy; to discard such an objection with melodramatic outrage and vitriol. This would be the temper of Platonism and may well seem quite in keeping with the tone of this book. To tow that line, however, would undoubtedly press this view of philosophy and poetry into an untenably ferocious ethical and metaphysical position. Such poetry, we would be bound to say, is valueless because it teaches no values, it is evil because it does not fight for The Good and if you're not on our side then you are on theirs! This, though, is the voice of the crusade and its clamour is impervious; and if there is anything which the philosophical ear must be, it is pervious.

To answer the charge of creation for its own sake, of merely entertaining stories, it will be necessary to say something about bad art.

A work of art (and specifically what is here called story, myth, or poetry) can be viewed as non-philosophical in a wide variety of ways, and it will be important not to create some sort of straw man out of very strong Nietzschean views which fit neatly into the anti-relativist stance of this discussion. Perhaps the strongest view ('strong' in persuasiveness, 'weak' in a technical sense) against which this present mytho-philosophy can contend with is some form of what is sometimes called 'moderate autonomism'.[11] This view is simply that artworks can possess a variety of different virtues or qualities and that these qualities needn't interfere with one another although they may. So a work of art may indeed have what has here been called philosophical content and it may also have aesthetic value but it may be that these qualities of the artwork have no particular bearing on one another. The moral value of the piece is not the reason it is beautiful nor is its beauty the reason it is morally instructive. The moderation of this view can allow for the converse to be the case (that the moral value does influence the aesthetic and vice versa) but merely states that *this need not be so*. This view appeals intuitively to those who enjoy artworks of an apparently dubious moral character (or outright repugnant moral character).

Wagner is a classic. I enjoy Wagner's operas less because he and his operas were tied up with, and sympathetic to, an anti-semitic movement in 19th century Europe which ended very, very badly. When I express diminished enjoyment I am often confronted with an indignation which seems to regard this reduction in enjoyment as almost tantamount to a logical fallacy; perhaps some sort of ad hominem aesthetic process. 'What has his anti-semitism got to do with how beautiful his music is?' I will be asked. 'Probably not much', I will reply, 'but a little nonetheless'.

My response to those who question my (slight) condemnation of Wagner is described by Berys Gaut as 'Ethicism' (Gaut 2001, pp. 182–183). This is the suggestion that moral qualities do (of necessity) inform an artworks' aesthetic value insofar as they are extant in a work of art. So a good work of art needn't be entirely morally laudable, but its aesthetic value will be diminished by its moral defects as far as they are defective. So much of Wagner is brilliant: the grandeur, the drama, the sweeping themes and deep, emotive character and story. It is also occasionally, and sometimes only slightly, a bit racist; somewhere in there, lurking in its guts, is something rotten. So overall I really think quite a lot of Wagner's operas, very much so (most of them), but I value them less for their moral defects.

I use the terms 'think quite a lot of' and 'value' precisely because they are *broad*. I do not say 'appreciate aesthetically', and I attempt to move away from 'enjoy' because what I mean to express is not precisely the kind of ethicism which Gaut describes. Ethicism is based in what is essentially a conceptual analysis which could conceivably allow for a non-moral piece of work which is nevertheless good; what will be defended here is what might be called a theory of psychological richness, or *'thick psychology'* which does not allow for such work. What is beautiful in Wagner's work is also bound up with that which is true and morally laudable in Wagner's work; were his work totally devoid of any such philosophical content (which would be difficult if not impossible) it would only be capable of mediocrity at best.

What I mean by 'thick psychology' is a view of the mind which considers it to be irreducibly complex. This is to say that reflecting on any given cognitive, emotional or otherwise sentient phenomenon in isolation, outside of the context of its other accompanying processes which comprise the totality of the person is naive and inaccurate. Once again, this theory fits into the broader theoretical trend of this discussion in recognising accuracy in both distinctness and wholeness. So, as before, what is not being claimed is a strong Parmenideanism but rather an effort in achieving a balance with more Heraclytean views. So, by saying that nothing can make sense outside of context, it is also important to note that nothing can make any sense unless it is distinct from its context: so individual cognitive states are salient but cannot be understood properly outside of their wider psychological context. Since, as has already been stated, this balance of continuity and discontinuity must be true of self and world as much as of any other phenomenon, this thick-psychological analysis of aesthetics and ethics is not contrary to a conceptual analysis but concomitant with such an analysis. This is just to say that rather than talking about how the concept of beauty must involve a concept of goodness, and the concept of any good thing must involve that thing also being beautiful I shall also (and primarily) talk about how the way we think necessitates appreciating the world in this way. *These two ways of talking are not altogether distinct.* Again, if we are the sort of creatures which must consider things in a 'thick' way (simultaneously descriptive and evaluative) then the world is such a place that it must consist of entities which are 'thick' in this sense.[12]

In using the term 'thick' this discussion follows the work of Bernard Williams (Williams 1985). But another important source of this use of the term 'thick' (to mean complex interwoven concepts and phenomena from spheres of life usually conceived of as quite separate is Clifford Geertz).[13] Geertz is critical of the artificiality of Gilbert Ryle's use of the idea of 'thick descriptions' and instead seeks to impact some genuine empirical weight to this idea by applying it to ethnographic work (Geertz 1973, pp. 6–9). My own attempt to employ this kind of terminology is in an effort to achieve a sort of amalgam between the ethical approach of Williams and the ethnographic approach of Geertz. I certainly mean to describe something on the scale of an individual mind, as does Williams, but I also want to illustrate the way in which moral meaning for that individual mind can only be made sense of in a wider context of 'thickness'. Ultimately the idea is that it is best to conceive of our existence in a morally orientated narrative-poetic sort of way and that storytelling and beauty should have a firm place in the pursuit of wisdom.[14]

What I am describing with 'thick psychology' is akin to universal synaesthesia.[15] This is the idea that those who demonstrate a remarkable conjunction of the senses are only extreme examples of what we all demonstrate. Some people might think Tuesday is blue, others that Rachmaninoff feels like silk or that a grumpy expression smells sort of cheesy. Some examples are more extreme than others. My own favourite is Ramachandran and Hubbard's bouba-kiki effect.

The question is, which shape is bouba and which kiki?[16] There is a temptation to suggest that some category mistake is being made if one identifies roundness with a 'boo' sound and sharpness with a 'keek' sound just as there is a temptation to suggest that a category mistake is being made if one identifies beauty with goodness or vice versa. In the case of extreme synaesthesia, there is perhaps even more of a disjunction between the usual way of seeing things and the connections being suggested. We are all used to thick moral concepts: repugnant murders or heartwarming heroism, and these are integral to both our daily experience and (as such) the stories we tell one another.

High degrees of synaesthetic behaviour are often connected with what is referred to as 'creativity' and also an ability to use the metaphor.[17] Of course,

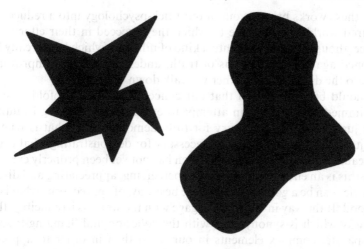

there is no implicit suggestion in any theory of universal synaesthesia that Tuesdays *actually are* blue or that the 'boo' sound *actually is* rounded in some way, yet this is certainly part of our thick moral talk and also common to much art criticism. Even if we were to take some very abstract art, perhaps the work of Mark Rothko, just colour and shape, it would still be entirely natural for us to talk about energetic or calming pieces, impressions of rage or pensiveness.

Certainly, as we begin to speak in this way, if we are not shot down immediately for pretension, the breadth of our thick-psychological interconnections becomes clearer, from extreme synaesthesia to familiar metaphor. It must be restated that what is not crucial here is any particular normative claim, that this piece of art should be understood as kindly or that this or that shape should be recognised as bouba, or even that one should find murder repugnant (though such normative claims will be made further down the line). What is important here is that it is entirely plausible, and indeed persuasively so, to suggest that when we engage a faculty of moral judgement we are also (though we may not be altogether aware of it) engaging other judgmental faculties of not only veracity but aesthetics and that this is not a mistake. We see the world in complex interwoven patterns and to extract elements of those patterns from that tapestry, to sterilise them and present their naked isolation as in some way essential is to misinterpret both ourselves and the world in which we live.

It might be claimed that the purpose of some abstract art is to achieve a kind of sterility, almost as an act of defiance against the gods of our minds, an experiment in human power. Similar motivations might be claimed of works which subvert moral norms (Nabokov's *Lolita* might be offered as an example) (Nabokov 1955), that such works are an attempt to break free from our natural inclination to conflate our experiences. Deconstruction and subversion would thus become marks of greatness and the degree to which these works bring us out of our thick-psychology into a reduced and fractured world is the degree to which they succeed in their efforts. This defence, though, drifts again into a kind of nihilism (which has already been cautioned against) and notions of truth, understanding and improvement fade into the distance the further we walk down that path.

It should be remembered that our concerns here are twofold: first and most immediately, this is an attempt to establish that talking beautifully is not just useful but necessary for fully demonstrating what is true and good just as talking truthfully is necessary for demonstrating what is good and beautiful; secondly (a matter which has not yet been properly expanded upon) this is an effort to establish that perceiving, appreciating and discussing stories can be a good way, if not the best way, of appreciating what is true and good. If the way in which we engage with the world is irreducibly 'thick' (in a way which is synonymous with the cohesion and 'hanging-together' of disparate, complex elements in our lives) then in order to appreciate any phenomenon in a more complete and accurate way it is important that any exploration is conducted in a commensurately 'thick' fashion. This is where the distinction between good and bad art is being drawn, between that which is rich and enlightening and that which is narrow and obfuscating. The same distinction is being made between good philosophy and bad philosophy.

Occasionally, stories for children are forgiven for being simple and unphilosophical in the sense described here. These stories and nursery rhymes may be shallow: nonsense songs and stories in which events simply occur, in which a two-dimensional protagonist navigates the most prosaic of happenings. It might be tempting to take these sorts of skeletal works as examples of unphilosophical stories which nonetheless are not 'bad art'. These stories, though, are frequently designed, and quite overtly, to introduce the very young to language itself and the basic elements of narrative and in this sense are chiefly practical exercises as opposed to descriptive pieces. Even so, it would be a grave error to imagine that stories for children need to be devoid of philosophical content. Certainly, it would not be controversial to suggest that good stories for children are rich in moral content. So, it is entirely possible to subject even these works, despite their seeming simplicity, to precisely the same critique as any other work. 'What does it say?', 'Why did he do that?', 'What happened to her?', 'What does this *mean*?' these are very much the sorts of questions engendered by these works in precisely the audience at which they are aimed. Indeed, even when a rhyme appears to be nonsense arranged just for the sake of entertainment, the very fact that its content is nonsensical and plays with our ideas of what makes sense and what does not is itself indicative of a quite significant philosophical problem. Reaching the boundaries of cohesion and meaningful language is a philosophical issue on which this book has already dwelt.

Hey, diddle, diddle.

If very abstract art and very simple art can both be criticized on the basis of their philosophical content (which is to say the manner in which they evoke, challenge and embody complex and broad concepts and ways of life in an effort to communicate a truth) then it seems fair to suggest that all art when it does what it should, is philosophical. As Marcia Muelder Eaton (2001, p. 211) suggests: 'Bad art is mindless and dulls the senses; good art demands, deserves and repays sustained attention, no matter what the community or traditions'.[18]

Of course, saying that art should be philosophical is not the same thing as saying that philosophy should be artistic. If, though, it is correct to suggest that the reason good art must be philosophical is that we experience the world in such a 'joined-up' way that philosophical art is both more fulfilling and better able to illuminate goodness, truth or beauty, then there may be a good reason to believe good philosophy must also be artistic.

It is important to emphasise that this idea of a rich, thought-provoking art being the best art is not a theory of instrumental good. Certainly, this idea of thick psychology does translate into a kind of satisfaction when one is presented with rich, complex, balanced wholes as opposed to isolated fragments of concept or form. This experiential 'fulfilment' is not, however, the primary reason for suggesting that this art is better than the 'mindless' art which Muelder refers to. Certainly, the goodness of such art is connected with this fulfilment but not dependent upon it; rather, the converse is true. Indeed, this is precisely the relationship between εὐδαιμονία and goodness hitherto discussed. It is useful to pivot this idea of art upon its intrinsic value because it is easy to recognise the same value in philosophy.

The activity of philosophy is good because it leads us towards truth or goodness, a work of philosophy (perhaps a written work) is good insofar as it demonstrates this truth or goodness. It would be misleading to construe philosophy as *good because it is good for us, rather it is good because it is an attempt to be good.* Nor would it seem right to suggest that a poem is good or not on the basis of the enjoyment it brings to this or that person. This thought mirrors the suggestions of Susan Wolf in her own discussion of the link between philosophy and art in this regard:

> If the source of an object's value lies in its capacity to benefit someone, it's value full-stop is conditional upon the value of the beneficiary. But this does not seem to be the case with art or philosophy. The value of a beautiful poem or symphony does not seem to depend upon our judgement of the worthiness of its audience.
>
> (Wolf 2015, p. 75)

By suggesting, then, that we possess a psychological predisposition to appreciate meaning and form in inextricably interwoven complex arrangements of concepts, sensations and impressions which are contiguous with everything else we apprehend, I am not merely attempting to set out a reason for the inevitability of art's philosophy and philosophy's art. This is not a brief psychological description of how we enjoy things but rather an attempt to point at why a more moral and illuminating poem is more beautiful and a more beautiful philosophy leads to greater wisdom.

Let's return to the image of the blind men and the elephant. With each additional aspect, each new perspective, the picture becomes more complete. Let's imagine, instead of that these men are not blind but merely very short-sighted and that one man, ever so gradually, begins to regain his full power of sight. At first, a trunk may seem an incongruous addition to tusks, and this vast grey side would seem an endless, alien thing compared to that familiar ivory smoothness. But it all adds up and the voices of other elephant-explorers, which had hitherto seemed so erroneous, begin to make sense, though their continued isolation appears all the more tragic.

We do indeed perceive the world as a rich and contiguous mixture of meanings and identities but very frequently it is that which is closest to hand and most sharply in focus to which we cling. The shadows of other parts of the elephant seem confusing in their gloomy vagueness, perhaps we can think of them in isolation but to allow them to encroach upon our crisp and solid world of tusks would be too much to take. Then again, when we think about it, these tusks move in unison with that grey mass, the subtle motions match the rhythm of that background breath. Our awareness of the world as a whole is certainly not inevitable, indeed, as has already been said in regards to the wisdom of the gods which Socrates was forced to deny, such complete wisdom is inhuman. Yet one sphere does, at least to some extent, inevitably bleed into another, rumours of moral judgement echo through our descriptions and a delicate scent of aesthetic scrutiny suffuses our logic. Kindness and cleverness are conjoined, though the point of contact may not be obvious.

This thick-psychology is, then, just another way of talking about the epistemic and ethical holism hitherto set out in relation to both the 'middle way' and 'living-with', by which a consilience of knowledge can be achieved and thus a state of wisdom attained. Without denying the reality and usefulness of particularity and focus, the effort is one of painting a plausible image of our mind and world which is cohesive and real, bounded not only by logic but also by ethics and aesthetics.

Art is bad when it is empty, when it expresses a paucity of meaning and significance. Stories are bad when they don't say important things because we are creatures who live in a world in which even the seemingly mundane is pivoted about matters of very great significance. This is to echo Murdoch's earlier point regarding Socrates and the peasant. The lumberjack and accountant may seem only to be chopping wood and checking numbers but they are creatures with history and vital questions. Any given moment of their lives is defined by every other moment, each impression only a fragment of an interconnected movement through time, primary and secondary qualities alike. As we perceive these people through media both critical and expressive, through languages of analysis and of evocation, our understanding will become correspondingly richer and more accurate. This is what Marcus Aurelius means when he explains:

> ὥστε, εἴ τις ἔχει πάθος καὶ ἔννοιαν βαθυτέραν πρὸς τὰ ἐν τῷ ὅλῳ γινόμενα, σχεδὸν οὐδὲν οὐχὶ δόξει αὐτῷ καὶ τῶν κατ᾽ ἐπακολούθησιν συμβαινόντων ἡδέως πως διασυνίστασθαι. οὗτος δὲ καὶ θηρίων ἀληθῆ χάσματα οὐχ ἧσσον ἡδέως ὄψεται ἢ ὅσα γραφεῖς καὶ πλάσται μιμούμενοι δεικνύουσιν, καὶ γραὸς καὶ γέροντος ἀκμήν τινα καὶ ὥραν καὶ τὸ ἐν παισὶν ἐπαφρόδιτον τοῖς ἑαυτοῦ σώφροσιν ὀφθαλμοῖς ὁρᾶν δυνήσεται· καὶ πολλὰ τοιαῦτα οὐ παντὶ πιθανά, μόνῳ δὲ τῷ πρὸς τὴν φύσιν καὶ τὰ ταύτης ἔργα γνησίως ᾠκειωμένῳ προσπεσεῖται.

> And so, if a man has sensibility and a deeper insight into the work-ings of the universe, scarcely anything, though it exist only as a second-ary consequence to something else, but will seem to him to form in its own way a pleasing adjunct to the whole. And he will look on the actual gaping jaws of wild beasts with no less pleasure than the representations of them by limners and modellers; and he will be able to see in the aged of either sex a mature, prime and comely ripeness and gaze with chaste eyes upon the alluring loveliness of the young. And many such things there are which do not appeal to everyone, but will come to him alone who is genuinely intimate with nature and her works.

> (Aurelius, *Mediatations*, §3:2:3)

Objects (and here Marcus Aurelius writes particularly of creatures) when viewed in a very broad context (temporal, spatial, psychological, ideologi-cal, biological, social, etc.) come, in some sense, to share in the significance of the whole. It is once again an expression of the paradox of whole and part: that the true significance of individual identity is expressed most fully when understood in the context of which that phenomenon is a part. Art which fails to capture this potential significance fails to permit something to stand out, let it speak, situate it just so with a flourish, a movement, a form; art which fails in this regard will only ever be prosaic in the most mundane of ways, not really art at all.

So bad art and bad philosophy are bad in similar ways and good art and good philosophy may also be good in similar ways, indeed, just as was stated previously when it was claimed that 'There is a singularity, a conceptually infinitesimal and impenetrable conjunction upon which our basic lived real-ities hinge', this discussion of methodological consilience suggests the same conjunction. As we draw out for a more general view of how we understand the world, the distinctions between art and science dissolve into a union of apprehension, of nebulous experience. Pythagoreans (and we may class Plato in their number) were obsessed by the parallels between mathematics, music and logic. Harmony in sound could be expressed mathematically and so too, to their wonder, could harmony in deduction and argument. An excitement over nearing some kind of core to the universe is palpable in that antique philosophy. Perhaps some part of that enthusiasm (though we might forgo quite its full extent) can pervade an approach to philosophy which allows for a more fluid methodology, where truths are presented both analytically *and* poetically.

But what kind of poetry?

Narrative, possible worlds and representation

It is now necessary to get a bit more specific about the sort of poetry which is being discussed here, in particular the role of narrative and how this fits into this model of pursuit of wisdom.

Discussing art in a very general sense leaves open the possibility of this broad contextual psychology, epistemology, metaethics or ontology as being a static thing. Of course, the idea of change has already been discussed and the necessity of temporality as part of this network of meaning has been noted, but even this might suggest something chaotic and amorphous. From the discussion of the idea of wisdom taken from the apology and Nicomachean ethics, through the ideas of betweenness and anthropological consilience and into this discussion of art and thick psychology, it might be imagined that this theory of wisdom rests on something very closely resembling process ontology.

In some ways, perhaps many ways, identifying the theories and methods hitherto set out in this discussion as being process philosophy would be accurate. The assertion of difference and similarity, identity and change, universal and particular as being interdependent and paradoxically coextensive does, to some extent, fit well with an ontology which asserts a theory of anti-substance monism. This synergy is even more notable when this anti-substance consists of what might be called process, being, experience or (and particularly) relation or 'to-do-with-ness'; things which pivot about 'actual occasions' as the atoms of reality. In the words of Whitehead, the world is composed of 'drops of experience, complex and interdependent' (Whitehead 1929, §1:2:1). Each thing is what it is *in relation to* other things, not by dint but *as such*. This is an attractive schema in which to situate this current discussion but has been bypassed in its more complete forms for three main reasons. In order to better clarify the model of philosophy and reality being discussed here, it will be useful to briefly relate these reasons and (albeit in a fairly superficial way) situate this current theory in relation to process philosophy.

- Firstly (the least pressing of the three reasons), there is a tendency to conflate the Heraclytean model in which identity is in some sense illusory or at least secondary with this Whitehead-Hartshorne tradition in which identity can and does take a central ontological place. Whilst this latter model has come to take the principal role in characterising process ontologies, this conflation is symptomatic of the vast range of theories (complementary and otherwise) which march under the banner of 'process'. This potential confusion simply means that any invocation must be accompanied by a substantial clarification which, in this instance, would not serve the discussion enough to be indulged.

- Secondly (and perhaps somewhat convolutedly), process philosophy frequently takes the form of metaphysical theory. Some effort has already been made to set the metaphysical boundaries of this current discussion. Whilst it has not been claimed (and will not be) that metaphysical speculation is invalid, the emphasis of this treatment of wisdom has been on the linguistic and psychological (and one might even be tempted to say phenomenological) foundations for understanding 'our world' as being the way it is. This does not preclude the possibility of supplementary metaphysical speculation, rather it simply focuses its efforts elsewhere in the hope of avoiding some of the 'mess' or risks associated with metaphysics. It should be noted, however (and here is the convoluted bit), that what has been called 'ontology' has been indulged to some extent and that the distinction between metaphysical and ontological theories is far from clear.[19] So some of the mess of metaphysics has inevitably and willingly been accrued through the (albeit tentative and sparing) invocation of 'ontology'. It would perhaps be simplest to say that the way 'ontology' has been used here is to indicate questions of *how* things are as opposed to *what* or *why* things are. This is to favour the more Heideggerian tradition of discussing the preconditions of anything rather than what that anything consists of, 'Being' as opposed to 'beings' (Heidegger 1927). In regards to process philosophy, this distinction may, however, be on fairly shaky ground, given that here particulars do, in a sense, consist of their preconditions (any actual occasion is what it is to other actual occasions and there are no other phaenomena or conditions). Suffice to say, that the emphasis of this discussion is not 'what there is' but rather 'how we should relate to what there is'. Evidently some concern with 'what there is' is necessary but is nonetheless of secondary concern.
- Following from the concern of metaphysical focus and closely related is the primary departure from process philosophy: Goodness and God. The theory of wisdom offered here has as its fulcrum an idea of the possibility of goodness. It may well be that Whitehead's God would (perhaps in great part) mesh with this idea of possible goodness quite happily, and the theories of creation and poetry to be put forward shortly might also go further to solidify this bond but that must be a work for another day. The intrusion of a pseudo-Platonic moral realism into such a well-established philosophy of substance

and change represents an addendum far too ambitious and tangential to be pursued here. Doubtless, there are those who would read this present species of moral realism, seated as it is in Plato and a hybrid Zen-Chestertonian anti-logic, as being identical with theology. I have left God out of it on purpose. God makes people angry. This violent reaction may lack justice and philosophical soundness yet I will try to complete my task without invoking divinity as far as I may. The field of Philosophy as a Way of Life (if it can even be called a 'field') already suffers from rejections by association with 'that God person'.[20] The extent to which debate about Whithead's God can become heated is also a breed of chaos which this book can do without.[21] More than this danger, however, there is the matter of what a theory of moral realism adds to an idea of a cosmos composed of processes, and this is a matter of *direction*. Oughts and shoulds are, as has already been suggested, built into the fabric of reality in the sense that they are part of what grants any event meaning, but they are also what knits any given actual occasion to the next, what permits us to make sense of things, and it is this which must be the focus of this current discussion of the 'poetry of the universe'.

So, it will pay to have process floating in the background but no more than that, it certainly is a philosophy to which this book is indebted but rather less so than to the theories which both this discussion and those of process philosophies draw in common (I mean here primarily the Greek conundrums of substance and change already mentioned frequently).

Given the cognitive stance of this book (that moral statements do make claims about the world and reflect possible beliefs) it follows quite naturally that poetry occupies a similarly indicative realm. This is not, of course, to deny the rich and diverse ways in which ethical and aesthetic matters can and are thought about, in fact, it is quite the reverse. Whether it is in terms of thick-psychology or just by highlighting the complexities of poetic and ethical language, this discussion is an effort in emphasising the endlessly deep and rich nature of our world. This richness does not, however, preclude *meaning* or what might be called 'orientation', indeed it presupposes it.

Philosophy and poetry both say: 'Here! Here is a possible world, what do you think of it? Does it not seem right? Does it not move well? Does it not mesh? Does it not chime? Does it not cohere and hang together? Take it up and make it yours!'. Philosophy sings this indicative song and its harmonies are played out in the consistency of logic. Contradictions and presuppositions are curtailed in an effort to achieve lasting structures, solid and graceful. The songs of songs, of poetry and other word art, are far more subtle in their mechanisms of power. It may be cadence, it may be tone, allusions and thick webbings of connections and interconnections of meaning create a dance with unfolding layers; yet, so too is harmony sought. As has already been said, philosophers can be guilty of becoming overly fond of their consistency, the neatness of their endeavour. Untidy edges, boundaries and axioms, are glossed over or ignored in the hope they might vanish in obscurity; paradoxes and impenetrable horizons are scorned for their inescapable power. Yet each song, each dance, each movement, whichever school or tradition, each one asks: *'does this seem right?'*.

Of course, this observation is a fairly trite one (that truth claims abound), yet there is a way in which the kind of poetry which tells stories (storytelling) embraces and illuminates the interplay of solidity and dynamism which this account of indicative practices necessitates.

It is a very familiar matter really; our appreciation of non-fiction writing in the form of history, ethnography and journalism represents a well-trodden path in the exploration of the boundary between kinds of truth stories.[22] Whether a story relates historical events or spins a tale of the imagination, each story will focus, will emphasise, will neglect and will move with a momentum of its own. Each element of the tale, however obscure, will be woven together with each other 'actual occasion' and will, together with its greater form, sing out with particular notes, particular meanings and messages. This structure of meaning might be called narrative, indeed, the narrative is a good word for it, and the work of Walter Fisher and his 'narrative paradigm' is certainly of importance here (Fisher 1990, pp. 234–255). As Fisher explains: 'the narrative paradigm assumes that arguers tell stories and that storytellers argue' (*Ibid.*, p.244). What holds one together is not so different from what holds the other together, 'cohesion' is a common principle.

Galen Strawson offers a particularly powerful objection to the trend of characterising both our psychology and our ethics as necessarily narrative in nature (Strawson 2004). Strawson is inclined to find a great deal of psychological content and activity in an extended now, and plenty of moral behaviour in that now too. It must be remembered that this current discussion of narrative meaning is concerned primarily with the *best* way to analyse and persuade, not a *necessary* way. The necessary bit of the psychology is 'thick' but not narrative, the narrative is an optional extension for gaining greater insight. So it is entirely possible to be not only human but also highly moral without being narrative; highly moral, but not *wise*. The suggestion is that those who do think in extended, complex and coherent ways about themselves and their world (in time) are inclined to be able to bring to the fore greater insights about what is and is not moral (by including more detail in moral deliberation it is possible to be more accurate). So Strawson's weaker claims are compatible with those made here. Where this discussion does depart from Strawson significantly is when he makes stronger claims of the following sort:

> ...the more you recall, retell, narrate yourself, the further you risk moving away from accurate self-understanding, from the truth of your being. Some are constantly telling their daily experiences to others in

a storying way and with great gusto. They are drifting ever further off
the truth.

(*Ibid.*, p. 447)

Of course, the greater risk does not equate to inevitable corruption. For
Strawson's simple, now-focused soul to be the paragon of ethical life, the
working conception of wisdom (and moral realism) upon which this discussion has been based would need to be abandoned. Storytelling may well carry
great risks, risks of dishonesty, risks of 'witchery and sugar'. Simple souls
may find certain virtues far easier to come by and to keep unscathed. Indeed,
such a conception of simple virtue, goodness as such, is important to this
discussion, since those (often non-human) characters are of vital importance
in informing our own quest for wisdom. But a perilous quest is nonetheless a
worthy one if its goal is admirable. Such stories are the greatest of all.

Why, then, not just stick to storytelling? Why talk in terms of 'poetry'
and 'songs'? The answer to these questions must point back to the idea of
'thick-psychology' and perhaps the best way to merge these ideas (of the
narrative paradigm and inescapably interwoven modes of moral, aesthetic
and logical appreciation) is through Rowan Williams' use of the concept of
'representation' (Williams 2014, p. 191).

In his Gifford lectures, Lord Williams set out to (amongst other things)
draw our attention away from an understanding of indicative language as
flat description and towards an idea of 'representation' as a more nuanced
thing (*Ibid.*). The distinction is a complex one but what it partly depends
upon is a characterization of language as frequently being a rich kind of
thing which is not simply a two-dimensional tool used to transfer meaning
but is, rather, bound up with the processes of the world. This representation permits a kind of depth to ideas, a living vitality or dynamism and
each word, each linguistic deed, becomes a kind of complex of relationships with the world. As Lord Williams explains: 'Rather than seeking
to stand in for what's "really" there, a representation is the "thereness"
of the object in relation to the perceiver' (*Ibid.*). There is no true division between our communicative acts and the world as an arena for those
acts. There are, of course, ways of talking, ways of thinking, which more
clearly demonstrate this kind of rich language. Poetry is probably a good
example. Through a certain rhythm, a tempo in the words, a poem might
evoke feelings of panic or serenity, words which at first may seem vague
are rendered powerful through the manifold possible relationships they
hold with ideas unspoken, even unspeakable. Indeed, each word and even
the music between the words is not one thing but many. Rather than a
cardboard cut-out, a descriptive word, dead and impotent, movements in
the poem speak so closely to the world because they are rich and complex,
perhaps endlessly so. A thought becomes an analogy, it becomes a way of
embracing the fullness of things more wholly, more truthfully, because it
deals in many media.

'Song' is a good word, let's use that, at least for a while, because the music of poems can be more obscure (though it is no less real). Narrative songs not only have a 'beginning, middle and end', not only do they have characters and causes, they also have another layer of harmony, of sense, of hanging together. The notions and words must fall in place but so too must each note, each beat. This is how the world is, how our thoughts are. Logic, aesthetics, ethics, all make demands, each one tickles our concern, but the end result needn't be a bitty thing, chunks of sense isolated from one another. Just as a song's words and music will fit, so too can good sense be made of morals and great elegance of argument. The manner in which a moral realism and narrative paradigm can cohabit is in just this poly-harmonic way. All that we say and do fits together as a story. Every object has a history (known or unknown) it has a type and character, every moment and person fits into categories of expectations which, far from being nebulous or arbitrary are, despite their complexity, woven together with the threads which we, our people and our world sow together. Behind it all there is *a sense of harmony as such,* and though this may be unfathomably more complex when it comes to ethical questions, the difference is one of degree.

> If our language is systematically indeterminate, incomplete, embodied, developed through paradox, metaphor and formal structure, and interwoven with a silence that opens up further possibilities of speech, it is a reality which consistently indicates a 'hinterland'; as if it is always following on, or always responding, living in the wake of or in the shadow of intelligible relations whose full scale is still obscure to us. To put it a little more sharply: these aspects of language seem to show that we live in an environment where intelligible communication is ubiquitous – where there is 'sense' before we *make* sense.
>
> (*Ibid.*, p. 170)

This is not a purely creative process, it is not just invention, mere rhetoric, it is poetry within a super-poetry. It is not complete, this is its point, each fragment of knowledge, though it is tied to the whole and defined by the whole, the connection stretches far beyond our ken. We may be reminded of the 'ἀνθρωπίνη σοφία' to which Socrates appealed in the Apology. This realm of analogy is our realm, the meaning is contingent and complex, flowing and deep, it is related to something less fluid, anchored somehow in its horizons, but that something is not 'ἀνθρωπίνη σοφία'.

Lord Williams speaks primarily in terms of systems of symbols (*Ibid.*), a very human sort of language, and whilst systems of symbols and proficiency with these certainly have an important role to play, there is no reason to confine this richness of interrelation to symbolic interaction. The ubiquity of sense would need to be open to the widest communications of interest. The kind of song which this discussion seeks to explore, the kind of story which it seeks to put at the heart of a 'living-with' philosophy is the kind of story which is inhabited, which is lived.

By carrying over the way in which we appreciate stories (in a way we usually think of as an appreciation of art) we can better conceive of how we should think about our search for wisdom in a way which embraces the in-betweenness which has hitherto been described in epistemology, meta-ethics, participant observation and, perhaps most crucially, philosophy. By 'living-with' (one might even say 'living-with-in', though that's just too ugly) a fuller extent of the meaning of each occasion, each moment, each person, each desire, each demand can be apprehended in its richness and the part it plays in grander wholes be better appreciated. When I ask the questions, how should I live? How can I become a better person? How can I grow in wisdom? The answer is first to listen, *to attend.* Listen to the song as it is sung about you, listen to its many voices. Attend to discord and cacophony, practice simultaneous distance and closeness. Drawback is to see the whole and attend with great focus on the details. Immerse yourself in lives as diverse as you may and discover what rhythms and melodies lie deep within. Do not neglect yourself in this, for you will find that each word of this world is but an instance and each character is part of a far longer tale.

Notes

1 This particular fragment is one of my favourites and is perhaps, for this rea-son, given a more prominent place here than it really deserves. Μονώτερος is variously translated and the fragment shifts significantly in meaning depend-ing upon how this is done. The edition of the Greek text consulted here is that of Rhys Roberts who translates this word as 'more self-centred'. 'The more of a loner I become' is also used and this certainly gives a different feel. The pas-sage of Demetrius from which the fragment is taken is itself concerned with the unique nature of this word and the way it can be contrasted with some-thing like 'solitary' (αὐτίτης). I suspect 'loner' does get closer to the meaning here, but I suspect it has something to do with a certain aloneness which per-mits one to have the space to give time to one's own thoughts. Either way, it is this state which Aristotle identifies as correlating with his increasing fondness of stories.

2 'Thus, the lover of stories is, in a sense, a philosopher, since stories are com-posed of wonders'.

3 This is probably just as useful as any shorthand for the sort of realism which has been suggested as being the focus of wisdom.

4 David Zarefsky's introduction to this topic offers a good summary of this view (Zarefsky 2014, p. xvi).

5 Whilst historical, exegetical and etymological concerns are not (as has been repeatedly stated in this book) the same thing as current function and correct understanding, they do heavily influence our understanding of any phenome-non and particularly philosophy. Philosophy, by its nature, is a slow creature and its roots are strong; whilst for some disciplines, two thousand years would be a long time, to philosophy it feels like only yesterday.

6 *Ibid.*

7 In pursuing this introduction to the idea of the conflict between (and identities of) philosophy and myth, in addition to drawing on ancient literature, I am primarily indebted to the work of Raymond Barfield (2011) in his book *The Ancient Quarrel Between Philosophy and Poetry*. Barfield's broad historical approach provides an ideal overview of this topic and is gratifyingly anchored in the transcendental, Platonist model which my own suggestions seek to build upon. Barfield also gives a good sense of the inextricable relationship between poetry and all Greek literature and thought.

8 On the possibility of Plato being the originator of the idea of this history of conflict see R. Blondell's (2004, p. 2) *The Play of Character in Plato's Dialogues*.

9 Eugene Goodheart (2009, p. 33) sets out some of the ways the New Atheists fall afoul of more nuanced academic reflection in *Darwinian Misadventures in the Humanities*.

10 I do not dispute that the 'Axial Age' (as coined by Karl Jaspers) was a significant turning point in human history. What I mean to suggest is that the significance of this period (when all of what this book refers to as philosophy seems to have been solidified) can be attributed to a quantity and longevity of work through technological, political and economic means rather than any theoretical, ethical, or psychological advance. In some respects, I echo here the thoughts of Jan Assmann in regards to the role of literacy in what is frequently attributed to cultural evolution during the mid-first millennium BC (though I do not wholly deny the significance of this time period) (Assmann 2012, pp. 397–398). I think Aristotle's suggestion that philosophy emerges when people essentially have spare time is to some extent fair (Aristotle, *Metaphysics*, I 981b pp. 14–26) and this probably has much to do with the boom of such activity at that time, but fending off barbarians and burning poo to keep warm only makes the dedication to wisdom more difficult, not impossible. When (and *where*) homes are warm and children are safe and well-fed it becomes far easier to take the time and cognitive space necessary to gain grand perspectives. One's mind needn't be narrowly focused on the details of immediate security, it can drift further away and take in a much broader stretch of the cosmos without fear of necessities crumbling. But in dark times there are still those who keep the light aloft. The books of Lindisfarne and Kells shine with this light. It is a basic incarnation of philosophy, crude even, focused on the basest and most stark virtues and truths. Such small philosophy, hidden philosophy, may indeed be more of an ember than a fire, but how much easier is it to kindle a blaze from an ember than from damp kindling? We owe them much.

11 For a good summary of this term see S. Bacharach and J. Harold's (2015, pp. 106–107) *Aesthetic and Artistic Value*.

12 This is to reiterate the previous argument regarding the role of doubt and conviction in metaphysical claims. To imagine a more distinct gap between the person and world or aesthetics and ethics is as useful as attempting to imagine a world of primary qualities without secondary qualities, shapes without colour... which is just silly.

13 Geertz was following Gilbert Ryle's use (though that is of less importance here). Geertz (1973) discusses 'thick description' in *The Interpretation of Cultures*.

14 It may also be worth noting that, in escaping Ryle's rigidity and artificiality, Geertz explains that Ryle (1973, p. 9) made the job of cultural analysis 'sound too much like that of the cypher clerk when it is much more like that of the literary critic'.

15 The idea of universal synaesthesia has been and is supported by a variety of psychological studies to date, see Johnson et al. (2013, pp. 16–17) *The Prevalence of Synaesthesia: The Consistency of Revolution*.

16 This image is described in V. S. Ramachandran and E. M. Hubbard's (2003, pp. 42–49) *Hearing Colours, Tasting Shapes.*

17 On this connection between creativity, metaphor use and synaesthesia see R. Gross's (2010, p. 78) *Psychology: The Science of Mind and Behaviour.*

18 The role of that which rewards sustained attention will return as a crucial (if not the crucial aspect of wisdom itself).

19 People muddle these two things up all of the time; I, for one, suspect that it's because 'ontology' sounds a bit more complex and sophisticated whereas 'metaphysics' sounds old-fashioned and religionesque; so people say 'ontology' when they possibly should say 'metaphysics'. I also suspect that even when people think they know what the difference is between metaphysics and ontology they'll have a very different idea from someone who is equally certain. On this confusing use of these terms see Bacchini, Caputo and Dell'Utri's (2014, p. ix) *Metaphysics and Ontology Without Myths.*

20 On this association between philosophy as a way of life and religiosity (particularly in relation to Hadot) see Joy's (2009, p. 103) *In Search of Wisdom.*

21 There is no shortage of arguments about Whitehead's God. For a summary of this see Heartshorne and Peden's (2010, pp. 81–87) *Whitehead's View of Reality.*

22 On this in particular in relation to investigative journalism see Ettema and Glasser's (1990, pp. 256–271) *Narrative Form and Moral Force: The Realization of Innocence and Guilt Through Investigative Journalism.*

Part II
Life

6 Purposiveness amongst living things as a focus of wisdom and the usefulness of fringe cases for acquiring wisdom

To be, or not to be: that is the question.

(Shakespeare, *Hamlet*, 3.1)

It is not at all easy to convey my sense of relief (I will call it a relief for now) when I first see my tomatoes.

Spring seems to have a reputation, amongst many, for gentleness and ease, but life on these little farms shows it to be otherwise. I would say there is no harder season. For those who live indoors, those who work in warm boxes, I suspect winter seems the cruellest of seasons; perhaps it is for some. I know that winter is cruel for many of those other creatures who live outside, it means death, but for the grower of vegetables, the keeper of animals, it is the early spring which is toughest of all. 'The hungry gap' it is called, the time between the brassicas giving up the ghost and the broad beans offering their fruits. From the end of February to the beginning of May it is not unusual for one day to be snow and the next to be clear, warm skies. The tasks of winter are steady and predictable, they are matters of dead and sleeping things, rocks and old wood. Feeding pigs and mending fences. Cold, yes, and frequently uncomfortable, but not much more than that; and there's always Christmas. But the New Year is austere and unpredictable.

Tomatoes are always my first seeds to go in. They need time inside, undercover, to get going, they won't germinate in cold soil and they need a good head-start in order to grow enough to make fruit over a long season. So, it is entirely usual to start tomatoes early on a windowsill or in a propagator. But they're my first also because of what they represent, because of what they can do.

I have always spent time on my tomatoes, worried about them. People sometimes return from a holiday in Italy and proclaim, with middle-class abandon, that the tomatoes in Italy are like nothing you've ever tasted here. They are actually; many of them are inferior to the tomatoes I grow. They are like little jewels in the garden, they represent what the garden can do, it can rise above the bland, plastic course we have been set, it can bring true excellence through small and simple things.

I live with lots of these simple things: many little lives. I say this in this particular way not only for poetic force but because the many lives with which I live are not only human lives, nor just animal lives but the lives of plants and all that makeup what might be called the local biosphere or living environment. Of course, in one sense this is true of anyone. There is not a human who has ever lived in isolation from all other lives. Not only do we require a connection (biological and social) with other humans (we may think most obviously of our families), we also live alongside myriad forms of other life, noticed or unnoticed.

There are, of course, many living things (bacteria, insects, fungi) which live out their lives unseen and yet in direct contact with us throughout our lives. We are biospheres all of our own. I do not just mean these lives though. There is a sense in which these lives, these invisible lives, are as distant from our own as that of a butterfly on the other side of the globe, we don't really *live with* them in the sense that we do not have an abiding and dynamic awareness of them. I do not wish to discount these little, microscopic lives entirely simply just because they are not explicitly in the forefronts of our thoughts, that would be a crude and overly cerebral characterization of shared living, but (as with so many things) they will sit at a far point of a spectrum, for now, the hazy fringes of a sphere (they shall reappear, at its core and in a new guise, later in the discussion).

There is a more obvious shared living at the heart of that sphere.

In one form or another I have always lived on a smallholding. It sounds a very grand and bourgeois thing, a 'smallholding', and so it is, I suppose, at least in the context of the country and times in which I find myself. I would like to say that there is another spectrum here, with smallholdings occupying a place further along in some direction or other from the small farms which have constituted the homes and occupations of people everywhere for a very long time. My family, however, are not subsistence farmers. Though they may know how to grow vegetables and care for animals, they are certainly of the bourgeoisie, so my hopes of a spectrum here, some continuity with a greater, more fundamental humanity, maybe moonshine; we shall see. My family are probably upper-middle class: media types, hippies at boarding schools. So there was a time in my childhood when my father cut the orchard grass with a scythe, and we would, come harvest time, cart the apples off to the mill up the hill in exchange for cider and cheese (that's what they make well in Somerset: cider and cheese), but we did not live off scrumpy and cheddar alone. One way or another, though, this is what I have always known.

Apples and hay, sheep and chickens, raspberries, medlars and eels. And it went further; other animals, injured or abandoned, were nursed and raised: weasel, barn owl, song thrush, swans; all these beside the cats and dogs. I suppose this sort of thing might lead some people to rebel, that is what we hear sometimes, that children want something different from what they have been given. I have always found this to be an alien and distasteful attitude. Neither I nor my siblings have ever shown any signs of rejecting this life with other animals (I do not mean to boast, I am simply grateful to my parents for providing such a life). My sisters may not have taken up the mantel quite so enthusiastically as I have, but they would never dream of life totally away from these other little lives, such a thing would be sterile and hardly life at all.

I remember quite clearly the dawning realisation that not everyone saw other animals as we saw them. It was not that this alternative view came from other children. Children, as a rule, seem to quite naturally perceive other animals as being sentient creatures like themselves: 'persons'. Whether this perception translates into compassion is another matter, but the idea that there is a very sharp distinction between humans and other animals seems foreign to most young people.[1] No, the idea that other animals were not people came from teachers and parents, possibly TV (though certainly not from most media aimed at children). The idea was not, however, articulated explicitly, it was simply the way in which they talked about 'it', rather than using a more personish pronoun.

What's been said here needs to be carefully qualified. Recounting some halcyon age of inter-species communion might give the impression of a kind of species blindness, dancing innocently through an Arcadian wonderland. The word 'person' may be important here; in what way are they 'persons'? In a sense, this idea of 'personhood' is just as simple and transparent as that Arcadian vision would suggest, in other ways it is far more complex. Both this simplicity and this complexity must be treated if any sense is to be made of the way in which a 'life with other living things' can be instrumental in, and constitutive of what small wisdom we people might hope to cultivate.

Binary 'creatures', analogue 'persons'

Let's be careful when we're talking about words. All too well will the teacher of philosophy know the inner lamentations (and urgent responsibility) brought about by students who are not sufficiently conversant in Wittgenstein. 'That's not what X means' they say with all the conviction of pre-philosophy. 'X means Y' they decry from soapboxes built from such sanguine etymologies that it can be hard to know quite where to start in dismantling them. 'Person' can undoubtedly mean 'humans'. Most of the time I think 'person' and indeed 'people' does just mean 'human'. 'Man', 'ἄνθρωπος'; these terms are undoubtedly species-specific terms. But words like this, concerned with the identity of our kind, which are so rich in history and meaning, and which are so ubiquitous in use, can present real ethical concerns.

The kind of language used already in discussions about non-human lives will necessarily inform how we are able to make sense of non-human lives as lives to be 'lived-with'. Certainly, 'animal rights' are not, as such, of immediate concern here but the discussion surrounding what is and is not permissible in our treatment of other animals is closely married to questions about what sort of 'other lives' these non-human creatures lead; that kind of question is of immediate concern since it relates closely to the question as to what kind of life we can lead *with them*. Can these non-human lives be legitimate and fruitful sources of the kind of participant/narrative/philosophical insight hitherto outlined?

The go-to analogue for animal rights is human rights. Speciesism is lined up with the other 'isms', particularly racism.[2] There are undoubtedly many sounds and morally pressing debates to be had surrounding this heated war of analogies, but heat can be a hindrance. The rabbit hole of arbitrary or significant distinctions, of genetic differences and similarities, risks drawing us into a realm of obfuscation rather than illumination. I have no doubt that the genetic differences between myself and another human are simply a matter of degrees away from the differences between myself and an individual of another species. So too, do I have no doubt that I am less devastated (and justifiably so) when a moth hits my windscreen than when I see the lifeless corpse of a human on the roadside. This analogy (of speciesism and racism), whatever its defects or pitfalls, brings forcefully to our attention the power of words like 'people' and 'person' for with these terms comes an inclusion or exclusion from moral categories.

Lafolette and Shanks are correct to emphasise that the question is whether the differences we observe (between one 'person' and another) are 'morally relevant', and whilst it is right that we should ensure that our focus doesn't drift from our central ethical concerns, just what is and is not permitted in the realm of those concerns is far from clear (Lafolette and Shanks 1996, p. 42). Categories, groups and their names frame the ethical debate before it has even commenced.

As with so much of what has already been discussed in this book, there is a battle here between those who perceive important continuity where others see a significant difference. If one does not recognise moral relevance then what is one to do? Part of the purpose of this entire treatment of wisdom and 'the good life' is to demonstrate (or at least suggest) that one good way, if not the best way, to negotiate these disagreements as to the (moral) significance of differences and similarities, is not to exchange abstract contradictions and consistencies but rather to experience (in a direct and visceral sort of way) the matter in question. The way to understand that a dog is a person (in a very morally relevant sense) is to live with a dog (particularly one who is very much a person). This, though, is to get ahead of ourselves and there is still a place for a certain level of abstraction; time to frame the debate: to find our words.

The use of words like 'people' is, admittedly (though only in part) an exercise in political provocation and in training. When my daughter has always used the word 'person' to be synonymous with the word 'creature' an invisible barrier is removed which for others remains. When I talk about non-human 'people', casually or academically, the conversation is punctuated by confusion and confusion can be the seed of new understanding. Discomfort, discontent with the way in which I have used words inevitably spawn some kind of interest in why I have used these words in the way I have. The idea of manipulating language in order to establish or reinforce boundaries between morally distinct sets is a familiar one. Terms like 'subhuman' have been wielded in the justification of slavery and genocide and the idea of personhood if it is not entirely synonymous with 'human', nevertheless creeps in through lack of scrutiny: conflation by inaction.[3] David Livingstone Smith attempts to use the terms 'person' and 'human' to distinguish between what seems to be human and what is actually human. By this rationale, an android or zombie would be a 'person' and you or I would be a 'human' (Livingstone Smith 2011, p. 5). This departure from the philosophical and Lockean tradition of discussing personhood as associated with mind serves to demonstrate the confusion and moral weight behind this family of terms.[4]

'People from another world'. This is a comfortable enough phrase which may help to flesh out our understanding of persons and human bodies. There is no sense in which 'people' is being used here in a technical sense. Science fiction is a sufficiently venerable and wide-spread element of our culture now that this kind of phrase (though it may smack of a chrome-plated, monster movie, 1950s silliness) carries a core meaning of 'person'. Perhaps these people will need to be decidedly humanoid. The Martians of a bygone era, lurching from silver saucers, steam belching from unknown sources. Two arms, two legs, a head and, perhaps most importantly, a face and voice. Star Trek is well known for slapping some heavy makeup on an actor, perhaps an exaggeratedly furrowed brow, and calling them an alien. They are still certainly a person.[5] This might only serve to confirm that we do not use the word 'person' with genetics in mind, and it may only shift our focus from 'human' to 'humanoid'. What is interesting, however, is that people like David Livingstone Smith want to use the term 'person' to identify the moral irrelevance of 'humanoid' qualities since it is the observation of phenotypical differences which is at the root of racist discrimination. Instead, it is something 'within' which matters, membership of the moral category is based in psychology, not genes or appearance.

The alien is a tool, a shortcut, and certainly not my own. Mark Rowlands (2013) has utilised the idea of the alien in discussing animal ethics, in his *Animal Rights: All That Matters*, he uses the idea of alien abduction to explore the problem of other minds in relation to other animals (a subject to which I shall return). C. S. Lewis is, perhaps, a more surprising author who turns to the animal and alien in ethics. In his essay *Religion and Rocketry*, Lewis wields these dual ideas, of other creatures, terrestrial and otherwise, deftly and with comfort (Lewis 1958, pp. 231–236). Lewis is in no doubt about what characteristic is crucial in determining the 'moral relevance' of any extra-terrestrial life; 'Have they rational souls?', this is the question we must ask and this is the same as asking 'Are they spiritual animals?' (*Ibid.,* p. 232). This might seem an unnecessarily religious way of asking the same sort of question philosophers generally ask about other animals: *'Are they rational?'*. We may well suspect that Lewis, in his insistence on souls and spirituality, is attempting to negotiate the kind of difficulty those who emphasise psychology as the moral qualifier runs into when it comes to human infants and those adult humans who do not possess the usual kind of intellectual human abilities. Those who claim genes or appearance as morally relevant have a problem with racism and sexism, those who claim psychology as crucial have a problem with humans who do not match the intellectual standard. If, though, the flavour of the psychology in question were not one of abstraction or heavily cerebral cogitation but, rather, something less easily expressed and yet still somehow more basic and more immediately perceivable then our theory might be both more practically applicable and more closely resemble reality.

It is in an effort to dismiss this sort of question, of rational animals, that Bentham's famous quote is commonly employed: 'The question is not Can they Reason? Nor is it Can they talk? But can they suffer?' (Bentham 1780, p. 283). There is no doubt that the fame of this quote and its wide utilisation by people like Singer and Regan is justified.[6] It is the sort of morally incisive suggestion which cuts through confusion like a hot knife; it turns us away from the deep, dark box in which we have been rummaging furiously to show us that we have been looking in the wrong place all along. But do we ever ask this? Do we ever wonder: *'can* they suffer?'. I suppose some people do, they look excitedly to scientific journals which proclaim discoveries of neurological structures and particular kinds of nerve endings. This seems quite wrong, quite possibly horrible. I have never really wondered *'can* they suffer?', though I have certainly wondered, in certain circumstances, *'do* they suffer?', and far more so *'how* do they suffer?'[7]

Sometimes I will ask 'does it hurt?' and in the same way, I will scan the face of my dog or the twitches of my horse's back. I will glance up, when removing a splinter from my wife's hand, to check if it hurts, *how* it hurts. When there are fireworks next door and my daughter climbs onto my lap for a cuddle I will tell, not just with my eyes but with the feeling in that embrace, just what kind of fear she feels and so too will the dogs climb up for a cuddle when the rockets explode; I will read their fear in the same way. Sometimes, albeit rarely, I will wonder if there is any suffering at all, it will be so deeply buried. Horses are very good at this, burying their pain, sometimes they will just be silent, still, their eyes will be distant. More so, though, I will think about the depths of suffering, the nuances, the benefits, and, most crucially the *desert*. The kind of core to creatures to which Bentham turns our attention, the basic capacities we have to suffer, may indeed be basic in the sense of being ubiquitous and fundamental but it is nonetheless a dimension of deep complexity. We need a language which conveys this complexity; thick descriptions, true stories.

Merely pointing to perceived similarities in behaviour (physical or neuro-logical) which are analogous to our own human behaviour will do nothing to 'argue' for the kind of concern and insight which is crucial to our sense of other living things as capable of pain or any other state which is constitutive of being a person. Any point of similarity can be emphasised just as much as any point of divergence. Moral relevance requires a far richer language which is already embedded in the morally suffused world in which we (living things) live together. As David Cockburn says:

> ...this point applies to the appeal to the great similarities between what goes on in the nervous systems of a human being in pain and of a dog that has been hit by a car. Certainly, this appeal *might* move somebody who had doubt about pain in dogs. But he might equally conclude from the similarity, and 'the obvious fact that dogs don't feel anything', that what happens in the nervous system is a far less decisive mark of pain than he had previously supposed. No doubt he would have to be crazy or corrupt to draw this conclusion. But then he would have had to be crazy or corrupt in the first place to doubt that dogs feel pain. The appeal to this 'decisive similarity' does not provide us with an 'argument' where before we had 'only common sense'.
>
> (Cockburn 1994, pp. 138–139)

Perhaps Lewis' language of 'spirituality' can help resolve the confusion around words like 'people', 'rationality' and 'suffering'. It might be easier to attribute complexity to something like 'spirituality' than to 'rationality'. What I mean by this is that, although Lewis uses these terms interchangeably, we are used to thinking about rationality in a quite binary and Kantian sort of way: either you are or are not a rational being. Rationality is more like a simple capacity or potential than it is a realisation or exercise of anything. Quite possibly Lewis would say the same about spirituality (and we need not follow Lewis too far with this term) but the use of the word 'spiritual' is far less obviously binary. It is easy to imagine one person being more or less spiritual than the last and in quite different sorts of ways. I wish to say the same about personhood as such. 'Intelligence' might be thought of in a similar way and the temptation may be to try to find something like intelligence which helps us understand and justify the differences in our interactions with and expectations of and for different kinds of creature. Certainly, I talk to young children in a different way from the way I talk to philosophy students, I also expect different things from them and for them but they are all fellow persons, 'someones' rather than 'somethings'.[8] There is something different in kind about the qualities which differentiate these different people from one another and the qualities which differentiate them from rocks and mobile phones. The first set of differences constitute something complex and analogue, the other is something simple and binary. My interest here is in discussing how we can best make sense of the difference between humans and other *living* things being of the first, analogue kind and how there is no third difference in kind, only more differences by degree: more or less someone.

This suggestion begs two obvious questions in response. Firstly, what are the ethical consequences of accepting this theory of 'personhood by degree'? And, secondly, how do we determine how much of a someone someone is? The answer to the latter query has already been intimated and will continue to be expanded upon through the medium of 'living-with' which has already been discussed. The answer to the former is a more complex matter but of less concern than may be immediately suspected.

The question at hand presently is whether and to what degree non-human life can (and *should*) serve as the object of 'living-with' which has been previously outlined as a good means of pursuing wisdom (philosophy/anthropology/poetry). Can the business of philosophy consist in learning from the lives of non-human others? And, to what extent are non-humans 'others'? The normative corollaries of suggesting that personhood comes in degrees do not pertain directly upon either of these questions (though they are, admittedly, of close secondary concern). Typically, these corollaries, when they relate to intelligence, are imagined to be the sorts of things which are wielded in debates around human rights. If a chimp is more of a some-one than an ant then it seems natural to suggest that a young child is less of a someone than an adult. It then follows (it's imagined) that the rights of the chimp outweigh those of the ant and the rights of the adult outweigh those of the child. The singer famously answers this idea, that greater intelligence grants greater rights, with the observation that this is manifestly not true, that we do not think we owe less to the child than the adult (conversely, we may owe the child more) and this should show us that a lower intelligence does not translate directly into fewer rights (Singer 1975, p. 12). This is one of Singer's greatest contributions to our discussion of other animals, to have taken Bentham's insight and shown a plausible inverse relationship between intelligence and suffering (Singer 1979, p. 60). A world populated by innocent, child-like minds. Of course, Singer immediately acknowledges that accusations of anthropomorphism will be made, that any drawing of parallels between human children and other animals is simply to misunderstand what other animals are really like (Singer 1975, pp. 10–15).

Since the model of philosophy ('living-with') previously suggested is one of learning about how life should be lived by becoming familiar (through simultaneous observation and participation) with the perspectives of others then it is clear that normative questions about what we should expect of and for other animals are closely tied to our primary enquiry. When the question is whether other animals (or other living things) represent the kinds of lives which can reasonably inform this activity of attempting to live the good life, of philosophy, then questions about what we should expect of and for other animals come close to exhaustively constituting any enquiry into whether other animals are the sorts of creatures which can inform this quest for wisdom. We learn how to be good by living lives with others which demand that we ask moral questions and take moral action.

It is clear, though, that one of these branches of enquiry follows logically from the other, I must first at least suspect a someone of being a someone (more probably perceive them to be someone) before I can ask more complex questions about the moral category into which they fit. The only way in which these two lines of questioning would be entirely identical is if all someoneness were to be understood as belonging to a single, simple moral category or if the degree of someoneness of which a someone consisted were directly and in some equally simple way correlated to their moral category. The reason Singer's insight about the lack of correlation between intelligence and rights is so useful here is that, given the close connection between 'intelligence' and the psychological complexity tentatively discussed here as 'spiritual', it is easy to see how asking how much of a someone someone is does not necessarily translate easily into how we should treat that someone. Murdoch's mother of many children may gain more moral insight and the chance for moral cultivation from her life with simple souls than might the ethics professor who spends all of her time with other ethics professors discussing ethics.

I would spend money feeding my dog before sending money to save some refugees, I would almost certainly save the life of any bear before that of any violent criminal, but I may sooner prevent the death of that criminal than the death of a mosquito. These are crude intuitive illustrations, perhaps provocatively so, but they serve to illustrate the complexity of the relationships between the idea of personhood ('spirituality') under discussion and more traditional notions of psychological complexity like 'intelligence', not to mention filial responsibility and desert.

It is clear that much of this more traditional debate around intelligence does apply to this current idea of personhood. Some word juggling inevitably needs to be done when it comes to attempting to outline a relatively novel way of thinking about any issue (or at least one which attempts to escape some of the restraints surrounding extant ways of talking and thinking). 'Personhood', 'person' and 'people' do, admittedly, have so much baggage as to be likely to lead to confusion and whilst they may serve a political and philosophical purpose their conceptual viscosity renders them a bag of blunt tools at best (which is not to discount the occasional usefulness of blunt tools). In a similar vein, terms like 'rational' and 'intelligent' carry a two-dimensional, enlightenment-age quality which, though it is common to philosophy, still glosses over the complexity of lived realities in an unhelpful fashion. We are not isolated little nuggets of cerebral process which can be detached from the rest of our emotional and sensational lives; such a model, though occasionally argumentatively convenient, fails to stand up to metaphysical, phenomenological, psychological and anthropological scrutiny.[9]

Language, quite apart from being something which it is important to clarify and resolve in order to better express and illuminate these problems, is also a phenomenon of central importance in informing our understanding of personhood itself. Language as terminology as opposed to language as the subject in question. Language ability is certainly one key aspect of both the gulf perceived between humans and other animals and the way in which we think about intelligence more broadly. We talk, they don't. We think in abstract linguistically expressible terms, they don't. If you can't think with words then you can't think rationally. If an alien turned up and attempted to communicate linguistically, we would not hesitate to think of this extra-terrestrial species as a people. Of course, if this alien species descended from the heavens in vast machines we would be likely to have made our conclusions long before any communication took place. Indeed, as Spielberg's 'Close Encounters of the Third Kind' explores, our initial communications with an extra-terrestrial species may well be musical (or perhaps mathematical) rather than anything more typically linguistic. Evidence of technology and art seems enough to suggest persons long before words are exchanged or humanoids lurch forth. So, the language may simply be one indicator of what might loosely be described as 'intelligence'; technology and art being other possible options and if a species demonstrates any of these then we can be happy enough with them belonging to the same category of the creature as ourselves along with the ethical prizes which accompany that categorisation.

Similarly, we can well imagine tool use and creative activities being cited as evidence in support of animal rights in a court. They must think like us since they are able to do these things, so we should think of them as being like us in morally relevant ways. You have passed the test, welcome to the club! Nor does this kind of thinking seem to be in direct opposition to the Benthamite insight on suffering. Ideas about psychological complexity inform our understanding of suffering. If someone can think about themselves in abstract, linguistic ways, then they have more to lose and more to gain.[10] If someone makes tools then they can be robbed of those tools, of their designs, of their future. If someone can create art then they can appreciate art, they can be the sorry victim of bad art! Being a person because you are intelligent or being a person because you can suffer in a particularly rich way may differ in that one is binary and the other analogue but both may end with humans occupying a very special place, apart from the other creatures.

But this never happens in life. When I find my pigs using sticks to prop up their beds, when my horses kick the gate to make a noise to gain attention, when the dogs roll in festering corpses to perfume themselves or when I uncover the vast cityscapes of the ants beneath my tomato plants, I do not suddenly come to realise their membership of my group, the ethical elite, The People. If I removed the sticks from the pig's paddock, I have no doubt they would miss them, they would suffer in a way the chickens cannot, for the chickens care nothing for bedroom accessories. If I padded the gate, so as to prevent the horse from making a clamour, I have no doubt they would suffer a kind of disappointment, enforced impotence in a way the ants cannot, for the ants care nothing for dinner bells. The song of the birds opens a world of possibilities for pleasure and pain which is far beyond the cold, dark ways of the earthworms. But it isn't simply cumulative. There is no doubt that when the details of these other lives are revealed, with their simultaneously strange and familiar means and ends, our view of these lives is enriched, brought closer, but there is no tally which neatly matches a scale of personhood.

Certainly, the people from outer space may reveal themselves, who they are, through technology and art, and this idea can help us see the limitations of ideas of abstract linguistic thinking as the criterion for personhood but it may be the case that there is no single criterion for personhood. Tool use and adornment may be cited as evidence to compel us into recognising the membership of other animals in our morally considerable category, but despite the analogue nature of this collection of details: tools, music, communication, social activity; it is modular, detached and only half the story. There's no doubt that when I see the care with which some pigs construct their beds I am given a wider window into the depths of those lives and so too is the someoneness of those lives brought more forcefully into view, but this isn't evidence which I bring to bear on my deliberations. These details are part of a tapestry, not a checklist. It isn't that these things do nothing to show me that these creatures are more or fewer persons, they sometimes do just that, but they are only a part of a wider story of perceiving personhood, of perceiving *life*.

The force of Bentham's insight would seem to lie in a suggestion that morally relevant suffering is a more rudimentary thing than the kinds of things which are attributed to human, linguistic, technological and artistic kinds of psychology. The fear a cow feels when entering a slaughterhouse, the smell of blood, the sound of screams, these things require no abstract thinking and may even be amplified by a lack of ability to think in that way. Most of us can relate to the terror of childhood when the darkness concealed all manner of evil things and the way this horror has been subdued by an ability to think abstractly about the actual likelihood that any such monsters do hide in the night. If we become bogged down with a tally of language ability, technology, art, neurology, social behaviour, then we lose something of the raw and basic power granted by Bentham's turn to suffering. Something which is seen in the eyes, smelled in the breath, felt in the beating heart.

Demon tomato breath

Anyone who has worked in a greenhouse growing them knows the smell of the breath of tomatoes. My wife worked so long and monotonously in such a place that she can no longer stand the smell, to me it is still a smell of rare deliciousness.

'Breath'? Surely 'the smell of tomatoes' would do just as well, better even. 'Breath' would just be poetic license gone too far, obfuscation rather than illumination, a trick of words to bring the worlds of vegetables and animals closer. Poetry as opposed to philosophy. Sentiment rather than good sense.

Yet, if there is no sharp morally relevant distinction to be drawn between humans and other animals then why stop at animals? Surely the difference between animals and plants is just a matter of degrees. And then why stop there? If we're including plants why not rocks? Why not volcanoes, oceans, clouds of dust, balls of burning gas which sail through the heavens? Aren't these just lesser persons?

There are two initial concerns here: (1) terminology and (2) reductio ad absurdum. Words are like analogies, stretch them too far and they fail. Arguments from reductio ad absurdum don't hold much water. The latter problem may assist in resolving the former.

It will be important now, rather than continuing to trip over the persistent tangle of meanings of our blunt, rusty tools, to arrive at some terms which are rather less clumsy (1). Having outlined a starting point for the kind of analogue concept which is in question, something which is, in part, about personhood, someoneness, perspective and degrees of psychological complexity, but more centrally about something raw and basic, something which can suffer, it will be important to refine this idea further so as to forge something wieldier.

At the very least, the reductio sounds out the clarion call of philosophy in general: 'consistency!', and so we may be tempted to push this idea of something with psychological suffering towards something more elemental, something to do with 'life'.

Of course, we could always just ignore the reductio. I have already dismissed the bloody-minded, clean freakishness of philosophy before, with its puerile allergy to loose ends, and reductio ad absurdum is rather less reputable than the law of non-contradiction. Why be bothered by this urgency for consistency? I can dissolve the boundaries between two sets and reinforce the boundaries between two similar sets, why not?

But plants aren't people, they are not creatures either really, there is just too much about mind and psychology in those words, let alone the humanoid forms. By understanding why plants do or do not belong to this realm of philosophically/morally relevant consideration we can better formulate the ideas in play and their corresponding terms. 'Person' may serve certain philosophical and political purposes, but even those special purposes break down when they drift so far from natural language. So little remains of what we had when we began with these words that there is more confusion left than fruit.

No secret has been made in this book of the very short distance it moves from Plato and Aristotle, this present discussion is no exception. There can be no doubt that modern and ancient discussions of the life and psychology of humans and other organisms is rooted solidly in Aristotle's treatment of the topic. By once again acknowledging how and where my own theory conforms to and diverges from Aristotle it will be easier to negotiate these problems.

Aristotle is clear about the importance of grounding this enquiry, on the nature of ψυχή, in natural language (*EN*, §I: XIII; 1102 a28-30). Sadly, the term 'ψυχή' (psyche) has been heavily trammelled by modern academia and medicine, leaving little of the more nuanced Greek meaning to play with. This particular term has passed from the natural, into the technical and out the other side again, having been washed of its broader meaning and bearing instead the ensigns of modern medicine.

Crucially, Aristotle, as always, seeks to divide the phenomenon in question into distinct parts with distinct characteristics which in turn lead to very definite corollaries. The different categories of the organism have increasing numbers of parts to their soul, one stacked on top of the other (Aristotle, *De Anima*, §III: XII; 434). In effect, by disputing the moral (or 'living-with'), relevance of categories based on genetics, appearance, intellect, technology etc. I have taken issue with the modern descendants of Aristotle's categories of ψυχή. As has been a constant principle in this discussion, however, this sort of dispute (over the significance or otherwise of a category) is taken in a matter of degrees. This is to say that, yes, of course, humans are different from other animals and animals are different from plants, but the morally relevant similarities are what are of chief interest here. If I were looking to advertise an opera I wouldn't give much thought to designing a poster which appealed to goats; were I to consider where to place a fireworks display, I would give very little thought to the impact the spectacle would have on the surrounding oak trees but I would worry a fair bit about how it might disturb neighbouring dogs. Aristotle is adamant that thinking about ψυχή in its general sense is of little use in his own discussion:

> ...it is absurd in this and similar cases to look for a common definition which will not express the peculiar nature of anything that is and will not apply to the appropriate indivisible species, while at the same time omitting to look for an account which will.
>
> (Aristotle, *De Anima*, §II: III; 414 b25-8)

I hope it is not absurd to seek something more general in this case and if it proves that any relevance to 'living-with' is restricted to particular types of ψυχή then it would then be wise to delineate a category which suits this grouping.

I can only feel a certain selfish regret that ψυχή has been so comprehensively adapted and assimilated into the English language since it is clear enough that in its most general ancient sense it can accommodate the sort of phenomenon in question here. By leaving the term untransliterated we might overcome some of this stodgy modernism and regain something of the delicate, ethereal beauty to which Eros himself became enthralled.

Ψυχή does still seem less misleading than 'person', 'soul' or 'spirit' and certainly less cumbersome than 'personishness' or 'spirituality'. So perhaps we could attempt to wake ψυχή and not merely surrender her to clinical misuse.

A stated desire to revive ancient meanings does not, however, help us negotiate how we can get away from any instinct to delineate different aspects of ψυχή and render any general category less significant. If the only thing which matters to living-with is that a thing is *living*, that it has (as Aristotle might suggest) a nutritive aspect to its ψυχή then why bother with the rest? Why not just talk about 'life' and be done with ψυχή or anything like it. One immediate response to this suggestion is that 'life' can carry a very binary sense (life or death) and for this reason does not fit the model of difference by the degree which is being discussed here. Another more important point is that what is required is something which captures both quantity and quality; this is to emphasise the importance of accommodating both the way in which it is reasonable to say that a butterfly's way of life is *different* from my own and, how, in a certain strict (and morally relevant) sense, it is also *lesser*. What is needed is a certain meaning which Bentham's 'suffering' conveys but without the necessity of 'sentience' with its heavily 'psychological' flavour of awareness and reflection, and its tendency to take on a similar binary vitalism to 'life'.

It is fortunate that at this juncture that a return to the outset of this book is prudent, for 'wellbeing', 'εὐδαιμονία' is the stated goal of this exercise (both present academically, and more broadly: philosophically and in life). Things with ψυχή are things which can be more or less *well*, indeed, their δαίμων can be more or less εὐ. This is emphatically not a question of either physical wellbeing or mental wellbeing, it is something which necessarily requires dissolution of that distinction into a more teleologically orientated conception of wellbeing.

The idea that a tomato plant can possess εὐδαιμονία may seem just as fanciful (if not more so) as the idea that a tomato might have some kind of psychology. Surely one requires the other, you can't have εὐδαιμονία without a mind. To attend to this problem in any detail might seem to indulge might seem to veer dangerously close to becoming a problem of philological interest rather than one of conceptual analysis. Εὐδαιμονία, since it is so closely associated with wisdom, may well carry too much sense of a peculiarly human route to wellbeing but the important sense which it does convey is the way in which the wellbeing of those who have achieved εὐδαιμονία is dependent upon a kind of fulfilment of purpose, a *directional* way of being which is somehow inherent rather than a product of inclination. There is certainly no stretching required in order to think about the 'flourishing' or 'doing-well' of other living things and it is precisely this which is of uttermost importance in gaining wisdom through living with. Indeed, the culmination of much of this discussion so far is in the suggestion that human flourishing is only one particular form of flourishing amongst many and, what is more, it is peculiar in that it is constituted, at least in part, by the understanding of and pursuit of the flourishing of other lives.[11]

It might be suggested that if ψυχή has been tainted by medicine then δαίμων has been tainted by religion even more so. Maybe we would be best to abandon Greek altogether. The direct relationship between δαίμων and εὐδαιμονία does, however, lead to a potentially helpful role; its use by Heraclytus is foundational and its sense of being tied to 'fate'/'purpose'/'towardsness'/τέλος is of supreme importance here. Perhaps a more direct transliteration ('daimorn') could escape senses of ghosts and ghouls although we might wish to keep some of that anyway. Δαίμων gives a sense of that early time when Greek philosophy first emerged from stories, stories of nature spirits as the forces which shaped our lives. And we may be far enough away from the literal interpretation of those stories and of the fears of the early church that δαίμων could bring just the right kind of baggage to this discussion of the directional quality of 'living things' (that which means they can be more or less well).[12] What will be crucial to bring to my own use of δαίμων will be a sense in which it can come in degrees, in differing quantities: lesser and greater demons. As with the previous rational for leaving εὐδαιμονία untranslated and even untransliterated, so with δαίμων; if any rough English equivalent must be read in its place then it should be something like 'capacity for flourishing' or 'livingness'.

The relationship between what was previously discussed as personhood and what is now expanded to be the capacity for a purposiveness or teleologically orientated way of being and wellbeing, may seem distant cousins at best, if not entirely unrelated. If, however, some idea of τέλος, of purposiveness, were taken in a weak sense as central to both personhood and a capacity for wellbeing then this distance might be reduced to a point, to nothing. By 'τέλος in a weak sense' what is meant is that no grand metaphysics is necessarily implicit. One need not posit some grand design or even terribly particular purpose for a tomato plant in order to agree that it does, *as a living organism*, and as part of a group of similar organisms, exhibit a kind of purposiveness.

Of course, this current book does posit a semi-metaphysical teleology insofar as it rests upon a theory of moderate realism. This realism is important for meeting the kind of objection which might seek out the teleological foundations which can lead to a stronger synthesis of the purposiveness of all living things and, ultimately, the way in which we humans should live our lives. This is 'τέλος in a strong sense' and whilst this is the suggested trajectory of the current argument, it is not necessary as a first step, a weaker sense of purpose can get us some way without too much novelty. This is to describe two distinct projects of:

1 Formulating a perspicuous and morally relevant category whereby 'personhood' ('mind'/'psychology') and 'wellbeing' ('fulfilment'/'flourishing') are seen as contiguous phenomena, different in degree rather than type.

2 Articulating a compelling theory of life whereby the activities of all
living things are seen as grounded in some more metaphysically orientated concept of 'The Good' which is both 'knowable' and inherently
compelling.

Both require a concept of τέλος, of 'end orientation', for the syntheses they
seek. (1) Requires only a very weak, almost everyday sense of τέλος, or purposiveness: much of what constitutes my own psychology (both conscious
and non-conscious): desire, will, purpose, hope, can, in a commonsensical
way (rather than anything more strictly behaviouralist) be viewed as common with the actions of other animals and, indeed, those of plant-life. The
fulfilment of a conscious aim is eudaimonically (and phenomenologically)
contiguous with the fulfilment of non-conscious behaviour towards a goal.
When I wake up in the middle of the night and drift hazily to the lavatory,
my actions are not clearly divided from those occasions when I far more
explicitly intend to use those same facilities, (say, before a long trip). Even
were we to exclude conscious aims as too qualitatively different from instinc-
tive behaviour, our own more explicitly morally relevant 'flourishings' often
come in the form of non-conscious fulfilments (from the avoidance of pain
to simple actions of comfort and joy). To prevent a woman and her child
from breastfeeding in their sleep (about as rudimentary and non-conscious
a thing as one might attribute to humans) would be quite as unconscionable,
if not more so, as any interruption of plans, schemes or designs.

Project (2) entails project (1) but also a kind of union of τέλος which is
far less easy to digest, far more removed from everyday conceptions of 'end
orientation'. If we can swallow the first spoonful of τέλος however, the more
hefty pill, with dandelions and slugs conforming to 'The Good', will go
down somewhat easier.[13]

I was feeding my daughter. She is still very young and sometimes she
would rather forgo the solid food and go straight to the breast milk. Lacking
mammary glands I find myself in the disappointing position of being unable
to sate this particular penchant so, when her mother was busy, I would use
guile and charm to coax my daughter into accepting solid food.

In addition to not lactating, I was also aware of the nutritional value
which solid food represents (if only, at times, as a supplement to breast
milk). So when Myrtle (my daughter) did eat, and when she ate well, with
relish and amply, there was a peace, a satisfaction, a kind of deep warmth
and fulfilment. Her eyes would grow both distant and content, her movements would calm as she chews unfeasibly large mouthfuls and gulps them
down. I looked at her chubby thighs and strong, delicate fingers, each (thank
goodness) where it should be, each coursing with blood filled with the goodness of her food and, alongside a heavy dose of gratitude, I was struck by a
visceral sense of my own role in her success, in her growth, in her trajectory.

Between caring for my daughter there were times when I was back outside, back amongst the pigs, amongst the vegetables.

At the side of it all, tucked away in a corner of the garden, are two plastic structures which look a bit like green beehives; these stout pillars house the worms. Of course, there are worms everywhere, they are the race of beings which writhe in the beating heart of it all, they throb beneath us and churn death into life, they are utterly necessary. But these particular worms are *my* worms and, what is more, they have taps. At the base of the wormeries are taps by which I might draw off the liquor of their digestion, leachate, black water. The leachate is food for the tomatoes. I draw off the leachate, I dilute it with rainwater and pour it on the soil around the tomatoes. I touch the tomatoes, I train the tomatoes around their string supports, I remove growth which will sap the plant's strength and I weed around their bases. Days pass, weeks pass, all of this repeats. The greenhouse is filled with the fresh, green incense of those lithe, vibrant beings. These vines also course with blood, a sap which carries the goodness of the worm-water, and in the air, I can smell that process, that flourishing, and it is not just loosely *analogous* to feeding my daughter, in a deep, abiding and powerful sense it is *the same*.

Peace, satisfaction, a keen sense of my own role in the fulfilment of these other lives, in helping to guide their trajectory, *of caring*. A visceral and barely conscious sense of the ancient past which stretches beneath these lives and the future into which they are thrown (into which they throw themselves). An extended and contiguous thing, rich and alive.

In the depths of night, she breathes, sometimes I have to check she is breathing, I will rest my hand on her middle and feel for that motion. Some dreadful idiocy persuades me that she may have stopped, that the world might just have ceased turning in the night for no reason in particular (because, for some, it does so fickly cease), and so I must check, check that she is breathing. And I draw close to hear that breath, and I smell it; so sweet and full, so soft and new. Not like the belching boglands of my ancient guts, prematurely aged and abused, this small breath speaks of gardens within, fresh and simple.

The tomatoes are always young and always exhale this same air of vitality. But it is heady and quick, full of the vibrance of a short and fecund life. Prince amongst its fellows under glass, the tomato is in a hurry to live enormously. So exuberant and enthusiastic is this force of life, with barely a space between this growth and the sunlight at its source, that a gardener must be constantly attentive.

A vine tomato (for there are many kinds) which is left to its own devices will become chaos of leaf and branch with little fruit to speak of. Respect for the tomato plant, for its way of life, and pursuit of its flourishing and of my own, does not equate to a passive encouragement of its own activity regardless of direction or character. 'Living-with', 'symbiosis', is not just a question of allowing any living thing the freedom to move in whichever direction it will, it is often quite the opposite.

Negotiating this need to constrain and generally infringe upon other lives is certainly key to the process of 'living-with' philosophy. Indeed, 'symbiosis' is a good term, not only for the pleasingly Greek note it strikes in this already archaically coloured exercise, but also for the connotations it delivers of a close-nit and multi-species negotiation of resources. For these reasons and for the sake of avoiding a repetition of 'living-with other living things' (with its slightly clumsy vagueness and occasional demand for tiresomely inverted commas and hyphens), 'symbiosis' will be used in its place as much as possible.

Before, pursuing the more nuanced and complex negotiations of symbiosis, it will be important to consolidate these thoughts on non-human lives by reflecting on why these particular lives are a good source of wisdom in contrast to a large human symbiosis.

Wellbeing I know, very different lives and honest

Allowing for the continuity of personhood and wellbeing through a very general conception of purposiveness, allowing for this analogue capacity for εὐδαιμονία, why, then, would we be concerned with the wisdom which might be gained at the 'lesser' end of this scale of δαίμων?

Living with other humans, learning their language, conversing with them, negotiating their hugely complex social systems: expectations and prohibitions, surely this would be a better source of wisdom, of ethically orientated insight, than trimming tomatoes. After all, the very definition of wisdom with which we are working (however broad that might be) is anchored in Socrates' apologetic confession of understanding 'μέγιστον ἀγαθὸν ὂν ἀνθρώπῳ', a humble and critical attitude which is proper to humans, not tomatoes.

There are three kinds of reason why non-human life is an appropriate focus for this analysis of ethical-wisdom through symbiosis (which now might plausibly and more neatly be called 'symbiotic ethics'). As mentioned at the outset of this discussion, the first reason is (A) that this is an area of life of which I have extensive and direct experience. There are undoubtedly many forms of learning through living-with, so very many ways of seeking wisdom through life with others, but this is one I can extoll and reflect upon in detail. I have found εὐδαιμονία out there, I have found it in the soil, and in the trees, I have found it in my cooking pot and in my family's enjoyment of the food which lies at one end of this chain.

This personal insight should be sufficient to excuse an articulation of a particular means of achieving a goal. As with other points in this discussion, this is the 'weaker' of two points, the easier to swallow. It is not necessary to claim the *exclusive* validity of the method in order to claim *some* validity of the method.

The objection, however, that human life, by dint of its prima facie preeminence in δαίμων, represents the overwhelmingly obvious choice as a setting for seeking wisdom through living with others, cannot simply be dismissed. Since human life is, by necessity, the fount and fulcrum of this entire theory of wisdom then one would need a good reason to go beyond philosophical anthropology (even granting the poetic addendum hitherto suggested).

An initial response to this objection could take a similar form to that which was previously associated with Singer. Just as a greater capacity for suffering (or wellbeing) does not necessarily directly translate into a greater duty of care (we may rightly care more for the infant than the adult) nor does it necessarily directly translate into a greater or more easily accessed source of wisdom (wellbeing/moral learning).

However, since some link is being intimated between the extent of capacity for wellbeing, δαίμων, and the manner in which we might practice symbiotic ethics, a lack of necessarily direct relationship does not amount to a sufficiently robust defence against an objection based on the prima facie preeminence of human δαίμων. More must be said.

Ultimately, a stronger claim than 'some validity' is being made. Living with non-human life is a *particularly good source* of wisdom because it involves (the other two of the three reasons):

B – Lives (δαίμων) which are *very different* from our own and,
C – Lives (δαίμων) which are, in a certain important sense, *basic*.

These two qualities: (A) the degree of difference from human life, and (B) being of a basic (or fundamental) nature, must be dealt with separately although they are intimately related.

The first point (B) follows directly from the central principle of symbiotic ethics as discussed previously. The process of learning by coming into contact with other perspectives is facilitated by (and to some degree requires) these perspectives being radically different from our own. The man who holds the elephant's trunk will learn less from the man who holds the trunk a little further on than he will from she who grapples with the legs or ears. For greater completeness of vision, one must seek out those views which have previously eluded oneself.

Of course, this kind of thinking, this seeking out of radical difference, has met with justifiably stern criticism in anthropology. The idea of 'noble savages' who live lives so distant from those of 'civilised man', or of wisdom from mysterious orient are manifestly crude and shortsighted.[14] Geographical distance and superficial differences between cultures do not translate easily into a disparity of ideas, perspectives, ways of life and ethics. One could as easily find a radical difference at home as one might find it on antipodes.

And yet, modes of subsistence, environment and history can and do *contribute* to a pattern of difference, and so much more so does species.

But just as the process of observation and participation is a delicate balancing act of opposites and seeming contradictions, so too is the fruitfulness of difference a complex and subtle balancing act. The principle of balance, betweenness or moderation which has come to dominate this book (and will continue to do so) is of central importance in understanding the way in which the degree of difference between oneself and another life-form is not a simple and direct route to ethical insight.

Indeed, it would hardly be right to call what I witness in the life of the tomato plant a 'perspective'. With enough δαίμων, the way of life, the location, the direction and experience of a living thing might be called a 'perspective', an 'outlook' perhaps, or an 'approach' to achieving εὐδαιμονία, but not so with any plant. And the lessons differ accordingly. Sometimes it may seem that the simplicity of the plants, of their sedentary quietude, has little to offer, that the vibrance and personality (and personhood) of the pigs invites a whole new way of seeing the world, and the kale plants just... *grow*. The pigs relish the sunlight, the beetroots merely absorb it; the chickens lust for the seed, the chard just excretes it. The horses feel the biting wind, the trees merely bend to it.

Differences of insight, simplicity or complexity, do not equate to value, yet some common-sense limits must be recognised. The difference of the life of a pig from my own brings to me new ways of seeing the world, a different way of life, but the way in which our eyes, eyes so similar in form, function and character, can meet and find one another acts as a bridge which the garlic plants cannot cross. The difference does foster fresh insight, but only so much, and it is not the only concern. Similarities offer routes by which differences might be reached, a common ground on which novelty can freely play.

And what of moral accuracy? Won't I learn more about goodness from the virtuous idiot than I will from the vicious genius? And what of those who are neither vicious nor virtuous? Given the (albeit tentative) moral-realism of this discussion, wouldn't this mode of ethical enquiry be most fitting? That pigs break sticks in a certain way, or that spinach defends against slugs by these means or those seems precariously irrelevant to any substantive moral insight. It may well be suggested that the immoral person offers moral insight by the contrast they set up, by the example to avoid, so one's company needn't be virtuous to be instructive. And yet, it might be observed that immorality is not the same as the unthinking amorality of bestial survival. A difference in perspective and way of life is one thing, but it must surely be a *moral perspective* to offer any kind of *moral insight*.

It must be remembered, however, how broad and inclusive the sense of 'moral' or 'ethical' is in this discussion and, indeed, how it is founded on a classical understanding of εὐδαιμονία. That εὐδαιμονία (understood in a not *exclusively* psychological sense) is a meaningful and plausible activity/ state for a non-human organism has been suggested and so too, does it necessarily follow, that 'ethical activity' (in its broadest possible sense) is also a valid predicate of a non-human organism.

This breadth of 'ethics' is, however, inherently bound to the balance of difference and similarity. Indeed, one can (though need not necessarily) learn more from the virtuous idiot than from the vicious genius, and thus do I learn more from the courage of a dog than from the postulations of learned philosophers. Yet the lessons of the plants are subtle and cumulative compared to the brutally stark virtues of social animals.

Perhaps what is most crucial, however, in understanding this process of symbiotic ethics, is that the learning is not achieved through mere observation. The lessons I learn from the plants about how to be a good human, how to be a good me, come in the form of our interaction, in the pace of life which the plants impose on me, on the way I observe the passing of time through them, of the way their simple needs force my own complex concerns into a levelled context of nutrition and growth, of water and sun, of life and death. And there is an important sense in which moral learning can be most powerful when the lessons are not given by another's example but through very personal efforts and reflections. Being confronted by a simple, dumb life, caring for it, neglecting it, conflicting with it, can offer the most vivid opportunities for the exercise of virtues and vices. Symbiotic ethics is not like a lecture, in which a learner is fairly passive, it is a kind of joint story-telling in which all actors shape the tale.

The conceptual space between these vegetative lessons and those which exude from the worms is negligible, so too that space between the worm lessons and the aphid lessons, the aphid and the beetle, the beetle and the ant, the ant and the lizard, the lizard and the toad, the toad and the mouse, the mouse and the blackbird, the blackbird and the chicken, the chicken and the horse, the horse and the pig, the pig and the dog, the dog and the schoolchild, the schoolchild and the teacher. There are no tidy limits within life, no ground barren of learning, no convenient box beyond which the lessons cease.

Even if we were to grant explicit virtue some pride of place amongst the sources of ethical wisdom, even so, what δαίμων, what capacity, is necessary for such virtue? This is certainly a substantial question and one which will be continued in the following chapter, but supposing we allow for the kind of simple core to virtue, a unity in 'ἀρετὴ πρὸς τὴν κυρίαν', or 'κυρίως ἀγαθὸν' (Aristotle, *EN*, VI: xiii; 1144b3,6),[15] which was previously taken as our starting point, then this is undoubtedly disseminated well beyond the human realm. And when I see the pigs wallowing in their mud, when I feel the contentment rising and falling in their breath, and I look then at the dismay of a human ferociously rubbing specs of mud from their precious clothes, I am given a clear picture of virtue and vice; the ἀταραξία of the pigs is masterful, enviable and laudable.

The final justification for permaculture as an exemplary setting for true philosophy (as it has been understood as a way of life) is the '*fundamental nature*' of this life (3). This is, of course, quite a grand and vague sort of suggestion and must be qualified carefully. Indeed, it is in this elementary or fundamental nature of permaculture, of life in the organic self-provision garden, that much of the force of this book is to be located. Due to the pivotal role of this premise, a fuller exposition will need to go beyond any brief role it may play in initially justifying the permacultural context. What can be begun here, though, is an attempt to link this elementary quality, this simplicity, to the defining principles of philosophy which have already been discussed.

Humility, honesty, first principles, self-sufficiency, freedom from extraneous concerns, clarity through simplicity, this could be a list of principles for either philosophy or permaculture.

As mentioned previously, 'permaculture' can loosely be understood as organic gardening or farming. Other terms in this family might be 'homesteading', 'self-sufficiency', 'sustainable-agriculture' or 'self-provision gardening'. A firm definition of permaculture is unnecessary at this juncture, what is crucial is that this concept and its allies place an emphasis on the interconnected nature of the activities of the permaculturist. The end goal is not merely to create a garden but to live in a way by which both human and non-human life might flourish in tandem. We do not grow rhododendrons, we grow rhubarb, we do not tend herbaceous borders, we tend herbs; a garden without a kitchen is as alien to permaculture as no garden at all.[16]

Part of philosophy as a way of life as it has been discussed here, this revival of an original form, is an idea of disposing of or at least drawing one's energy and attention away from those aspects of life which are less vital. When Socrates challenges his accusers and expands upon the Oracle's claim, and (to a lesser extent) when he conducts any dialogue with those Plato sends his way, he is stripping things away. Preconceptions, poorly founded confidence, misplaced priorities, untenable inconsistencies, unnecessary distractions, these things are the primary victims of Socrates' philosophical fire. By paring down our thoughts Socrates helps to reveal the foundations of our ideas and our way of life, this is a process driven by and aimed towards intellectual honesty. Permaculture shares this impetus.

Now, whether a particular economic or political movement shares more or less with Socrates' (or Plato's) philosophy is: (A) not exhaustive of the wider aims and principles of 'seeking wisdom/wellbeing' which have been discussed here and (B) sufficiently vague that it may well just lead us right back to the kind of monastic elitism which was objected to at the outset of this discussion. Extolling the virtues of stripping away unnecessary distractions could (if we pursued it to its 'logical' conclusion) prescribe for us a life which, in Susan Wolf's words, seems 'strangely barren' (Wolf 1982, p. 421). Austere cloisters and silent dinners, a renunciation of belongings and an exclusive dedication to truth, beauty and goodness. Indeed, many people who follow the life of permaculture, who live with other living things through this delicate negotiation of shared resources, do profess a similar ethic of renunciation. Dismay at consumerism and a desire to lead a life free from 'stuff' grip many of my friends and perhaps there is some truth here, some good sense, but before we go any distance down that foreboding path, let us (as usual) take a less onerous step towards this 'honesty' first.

Quite apart from the consequentialist considerations of hugely complex and extended farming, processing, transport and distribution industries which are necessary to get food from the soil to a shop, and besides the virtues and vices embroiled therein, there is the simple matter of being directly acquainted with the whole process.

There are certainly more pressing ethical layers to (real) philosophy, but if we were to concentrate only on philosophy's conventional mission of perceiving and comprehending the more vital and basic aspects of any given phenomenon or concept, then permaculture mimics this principle closely in the transparency it offers.

I collect the beans from the bean plants. Some of these beans I eat, others I save and, come the next summer, I plant them in the soil and (slugs allowing) they grow into more bean plants. I eat some of these new beans and some I save for next year. This is the extent of things. Mere meters, feet, worms, dirty fingernails. Nothing is hidden, everything is directly apparent. It may be more visceral, more enacted, but the process of becoming directly familiar with my food is very close indeed to the process of becoming directly familiar with my thoughts, with my meaning.

Were I to exclude the non-human elements from living-with then I would be floating on a sea of lazy assumptions; were my effort in ethics to be practised without permaculture then it would be oblivious to the invisible lives without which it would not be possible. Quite apart from anything else, the organic garden is an effort in transparency, in illumination, and for this reason, it is also a preeminent (possibly necessary) setting for ethics. This is the kind of definition of permaculture with which this discussion is dealing. María De La Bellacasa suggests in her *Matters of Care* that: 'permaculture practices are ethical doings that engage with ordinary personal living and subsistence as part of a collective effort that includes nonhumans' (De La Bellacasa 2017, p. 145). This inclusion of non-humans in consideration of 'ethical doings' in 'ordinary personal living' offers a sufficient description of permaculture for the purposes of this discussion.

The beans from the shop are less philosophical, less ethical, than the beans from my garden.

Notes

1 Indeed, this recognition of personhood can accompany malice as opposed to compassion (*Cf.* Hurn 2012, p. 100).
2 Hugh Lafollette and Niall Shanks do a nice job of indicating the central (and expected) nature of this particular meeting of 'isms' (Lafolette and Shanks 1996, pp. 41–61).
3 On the use of language to dehumanise humans see Livingstone Smith's (2011) *Less Than Human: Why We Demean, Enslave, and Exterminate Others*.
4 P. F. Snowdon (2014, pp. 11; 58–64) in *Persons, Animals, Ourselves* discusses this issue of terminological departure.
5 It is only fair to note that Star Trek, being the bastion of pop-philosophy that it is, dealt quite early on with the question of animality (in its own peculiar way) in the film *The Voyage Home* (1986). Here an alien probe threatens Earth and speaks in the language of humpback whales and it is only they who can

save Earth. In a rather more intellectually sophisticated and satirical twist, we might also think of Douglas Adams' (1984) *So Long and Thanks for All the Fish* in which the Dolphins of Earth, far from saving the planet, abandon it prior to its destruction.

6 Used by Regan (1983, p. 95) notably in *The Case for Animal Rights*; and Singer (1975, p. 7) most notably in *Animal Liberation: A New Ethics for Our Treatment of Animals*.

7 This is one of many suggestions made in this book which are largely indebted to Raimond Gaita's (2003, pp. 106–111) work in *The Philosopher's Dog*. Gaita criticises a kind of 'scientistic' way of thinking about proof when it comes to how we should think about other animals.

8 I take this language (though it is natural enough) of 'someone' and something' from Robert Spaemann (Spaemann 2006).

9 Of course, there are very few (academics) who would adhere to any crude forms of ratio-centric mind-body dualism. Brie Gertler laments this kind of straw-manning of dualism and defends a kind of naturalistic dualism from physicalist criticism on the basis that physicalist objections suffer from worse problems than the naturalist dualist (Gertler 2005, p. 295). My own criticism is not, however, anywhere near a physicalist approach and is closer to what I have tried to characterise as roughly Wittgensteinian. It may also be tempting to describe the approach as phenomenological and I hope there is room for a conjunction between ideas which might more commonly be conceived of as phenomenological and those which might be thought of as related to *making sense*. On this conjunction see R. A. Noë's (1994, pp. 1–42) *Wittgenstein, Phenomenology and What It Makes Sense to Say*. Noë is more broadly concerned with an exegesis of Wittgenstein which situates phenomenological thinking securely within the development of Wittgenstein's work. My own use of the phrase 'making sense' and its cognates is broader and closer to the way in which Gaita talks about 'meaning' (Gaita 2003, pp. 95–115).

10 Raymond Frey is probably the best known proponent of using criteria of this kind to judge the moral importance of non-human animals. In many ways, the 'degrees of moral status' argument which I follow here reflects the utilitarian arguments of Frey. I do not, of course, follow Frey's thoughts on 'quality of life' in the kind of way he means something more like 'how much life is being enjoyed' (I understand it is not quite as crude as this but I mean to set up a contrast). My own scale relates to a thick concept of fulfilment in which being alive, *life as such*, carries a great deal of weight. Ultimately, much of the divergence here comes down to where the weights are placed. My own suggestion is that it is only through the kind of 'living-with' described above that these kinds of weights (on psychological complexity, being alive, being in conflict etc.) can be (more or less) accurately assessed (Frey 2011, pp. 189–193).

11 One might be inclined, at this stage, to give this key to human flourishing a name, perhaps the name of virtue, 'compassion' or 'love', and dedicate the rest of this treatise to the exploration of exiting theories of love and compassion towards both human and non-human life. This would be to jump-the-gun but is certainly of significant importance in what follows.

12 An even deeper philology and etymology of δαίμων might suggest an association with division and distinctness. David Farrell Krell (1987, p. 24) discusses this in his *Daimon Life, Nearness and Abyss: An Introduction to Za-ology* in relation to Heidegger's discussion of Heraclytus's fragment as discussed at the outset of this book. It is tempting to take the usefulness of δαίμων even further, then, and to find some sense of the way in which a living thing is

particularly distinct and that the ethically relevant quality of living things is not due solely to their purposiveness but also the extent to which they might be described as 'individuals'.

13 It should also be noted that, along with the general ethos of epistemological, ethical and academic moderation which has hitherto been professed, comes the acknowledgement that the more novel (or at least 'novel' in the academic context in which they are currently expressed) claims made in this book may be rejected by any critic whilst leaving the possibility of accepting the less weighty claims made along the way. I'd quite like it if you ate all your greens but if you can only manage a few peas then that's better than now.

14 Hurn (2012, pp. 50–51) discusses this in *Humans and Other Animals*.

15 'Virtue in the principal sense' or 'general goodness'.

16 Permaculture is, for lack of a better description, a 'holistic' framework; it is explicitly concerned with the ethics not only of eating but of all aspects of living. The suggestion is, that the best way to approach this is through the sustainable and local production of goods (food). On this way of understanding permaculture see K. Fox's (2013, p. 167) *Putting Permaculture Ethics to Work: Commons Thinking, Progress, and Hope.*

7   The inevitability of doing harm, the importance of feeling bad and the central role of honesty and courage

> Thou know'st 'tis common; all that lives must die.
>
> (Shakespeare, *Hamlet*, 1.2)

> To observe [nonviolence] fully is impossible for men, who kill a number of living beings large and small as they breathe or blink or till the land.
>
> (M. K. Gandhi, *Satyagraha*, 2:28)

But I still fail, still one of those competition eaters, slavering as I drift through the supermarket, sloughing packet after packet of plastic-wrapped crap into my trolley; neglecting my vegetable garden.

And yet no meat, no dairy, no eggs... those are not for me to take; too far, too high a price to pay, too much death.

Honour's little space. Philosophy's refuge.

Not for me to take.

...

At the heart of the following attempt to expand upon and analyse the ethical richness of permaculture is an idea of 'respect'.

'Respect', 'honour', 'dignity', 'integrity'. Close familiarity with the basic demands of subsistence (and with a possible flourishing thereby) brings a weighty and solid meaning to this family of concepts. The tension of life, of the constant flow of destruction and creation, death and birth, of desperate manipulation and grateful appreciation, this coalesces in an idea of 'respect' which sits at the core of wisdom.

When 'respect' (for now understood in a loose sense together with related concepts) is on the table, Kant's second formulation of the categorical imperative seems a prudent port of call.

> So act as to treat humanity, whether in thine own person or in that of any other, in every case as an end withal, never as a means only.
>
> (Kant 1873, p. 46)

It is with Albert Schweitzer's addendum to that imperative, however, and his thoughts beyond that, by which the following will most directly be guided.

> True philosophy must start from the most immediate and comprehensive fact of consciousness, and this may be formulated as follows: 'I am life which wills to live, and I exist in the midst of life which wills to live'.
>
> (Schweitzer 1923, p. 253)

'Humanity' ('die Menschheit') isn't enough; life, with its δαίμων (its will to live), is to be treated as the end, never only as a means.

Of course, from the mere fact of it, of life amidst life, of life amidst death, a first principle might be quite bleak, quite dark. 'The most immediate and comprehensive fact of consciousness', *the first principle*, 'I am life which wills to live, and I exist in the midst of life which wills to live'.

Ultimately, if this idea of life emulating philosophy, of living-with, is to take an idea of basic needs as its foundation, then one cannot ignore *competition*.

...

I like to eat eggs.

Eggs are so different from the vegetables, they are thick with the things of which I am made. I think I can feel the difference. I am like an egg, I was an egg. I can and do eat notable quantities of eggs.

Rats also like to eat eggs.

I would go outside in the mornings and open the barn door, every corner rattling with frantic claws and the chicken feeder swinging absently. One or two rats would decide to run across the floor for a better hiding place.

The nesting box where the hens lay their eggs would be strewn with shell and occasionally there would be an egg which had been rolled to the edge in an attempt to move it elsewhere, perhaps a more comfortable place to eat, somewhere away from the door which might open, somewhere away from me.

They are not safe from me.

I will not poison the rats. Poison is truly vile. I have seen rats die from poison; their slowly rupturing innards heave palpably. But besides that torture, it is underhanded, they crawl off into some corner where the only evidence of their death is a temporary reek. Poison is indiscriminate, anonymous, pathetic. I will not poison the rats because it shows them no respect.

I let my dogs on them though.

Of course, I take many other measures to dissuade the rats from maintaining their hidden hold on my realm: I lock food away, I attempt to make it difficult for them to take advantage of when it is out for the chickens by placing it in suspended feeders, I alter the surroundings and block up runways and holes. I spray various strong plant oils of which they should not be fond. But they are a hard, clever, quick and tenacious folk. My last resort is to unleash monsters into their world.

Mostly the rats get away, they are usually faster and smarter than the dogs, but sometimes they don't; it is usually the young rats who fall. With a scream, a short fight, they are done. But babies are replaced swiftly in the world of the rats. A quick world, a dark world, heavy-scented, boisterous, careful, clever, playful, full of motion and close company.

I bear the rats no particular ill will. When the rats find a nice place to make a home, close to water, close to grain and eggs, warm and dry, why wouldn't they set up their homes here? They will no doubt sniff the air, they will find that air filled with dog smell, human smell, cat, but not much fox, and good, tight runways in which to hide. A good home, relatively speaking.

When I would shift around the feed bins, when I nailed planks over runways, I'm sure the rats became familiar with the fact that this realm is also that of a human, a human with dogs, but that is the way of rats, they are 'happy to share'. Better to fight in here than fight out there. This is not 'deliberation' as such, I'm not drifting away from the broad idea of δαίμων into something more familiarly cogitative and cerebral in our language-heavy sort of way, no, that would be truly anthropomorphic (in a bad sense), but it is clear that rats do a fair bit of thinking, in a rudimentary but efficient sort of way.

I had a pet rat once. They are truly wonderful creatures, very like ourselves in all sorts of ways, particularly in their indolence and society.

But we are, in our small way, in competition. In this narrow arena, in this little world of chickens, rats and my family, I am life which wills to live and they are life which wills to live. Not 'survive', each of us, myself and the rats, might 'survive' elsewhere and by other means, but to live *this* life.

But they aren't being malicious or neglectful and most of the time they aren't even consciously infringing upon something they recognise to be the territory of another.

But sometimes, ever so slightly, they do recognise this: that this place is, in a certain sense, the domain of another, of a potentially threatening other. Even if this recognition takes the basic form of merely sensing my identity in this place, my smell, my activity, and realising that this extension of my presence and interests is threatening to their own interests, the recognition is still there.

I suspect that this kind of mutual recognition is behind lots of anger towards other living things. It seems more understandable to hunt a wolf with passion and adversarial determination than it does to chop down trees in the same way. It feels more personal when the rats take my eggs than when lice prevent the hens from laying. But as before, as with the spectrum, the web or the sphere of δαίμων, from the outer reaches of complex psychology through regions of more basic sentience and into a core and vegetative system of absorption and multiplication, the struggles, the negotiations are different in degree.

Mark Rowlands once again employs the extra-terrestrial tool to express the need to understand the degree to which the rats do indeed recognise the extent to which their activities infringe upon mine (Rowlands 2012, pp. 248–251). Rowlands is ultimately concerned with a broader array of capacities which constitute the capacity for moral deliberation, but the recognition of infringing upon the demands of another is crucial to this greater capacity for morality. Rowlands too invokes Nussbaum's concept of flourishing and imagines Martians who perceive the importance of recognising human moral deliberation as core to showing humans proper 'respect' (respecting our capacities that we might flourish):

> So to treat a hairless ape with respect – the fundamental moral injunction – requires that one understand its capabilities, and treat it in such a way that it is able to exercise those capabilities, and so live a flourishing life.
>
> (Rowlands 2012, p. 250)

This kind of reflection might suggest that the kind of continuity between living things which has been pursued here is contrary to this Nussbaumian (or Greek/Hellenistic) 'fundamental moral injunction'. 'Respect' (now slightly more specifically understood as a recognition of and action on behalf of the capacities for the flourishing of a being) requires a strict discrimination between kinds of capacity.

But with the rats, the hens and the dogs, our capacities for flourishing (δαίμων) and resultant demands for resources are mutually exclusive. I have knowingly and purposely unleashed my hounds upon this people; I have done them terminal violence. Just how a rat thinks about me and that which is mine (or whether or how the rat even acknowledges that it is indeed mine) is not what was crucial to this violence, to this clash, what was crucial was far more visceral.

This was not an opposition of minds, it was an opposition of guts. I wanted eggs, they wanted eggs, and all along the hens who laid the eggs are almost forgotten. The meeting of demands does not occur on a cerebral plane it occurs in the dirt. The push and pull of different interests, of different lives, occurs less in a realm of ideas and more as a sheer bodily collision. There is a palpable sense in which my identity is extended into those things, into the eggs, into the hens, into the farm buildings. δαίμων and identity are one; my character and my story. The tendrils of my story reach out and cover the hens and their eggs like great roots; they mix with the roots of the hens' δαίμων and also with those of the rats. They interlock and strangle one another in an effort to reach the soils for which they strive.

Perhaps most academics are so used to their own territories being infringed upon through a lack of scholarly acknowledgment to be able to get a keen sense of the continuity of injustice between moral deliberation and sheer biological force, but the lesson is also out there, written in muck and blood.

If this clash of guts is so bitter, if this is a war of sheer life willing to live, then why not just try to win the war? Is this the moral lesson from symbiotic ethics: that εὐδαιμονία is to be found in brutal biological dominance? Is the ultimate wisdom and fulfillment of human life simply that of domination?

Athena: God of war

Some differences in the intrinsic value of living things have already been suggested as plausible, and an attempt has been made at characterising these differences as non-dualistic and not purely psychological through the idea of δαίμων. Some account must, therefore, be made of how any normative positions regarding non-human life are affected by this idea.

If it were suggested that all life were in some way equally valuable, if it were acknowledged that complex psychology and even psychology as such were not necessary conditions for intrinsic value, but that the intrinsic value was of a single undifferentiated kind, then the moral conundrums would be of a particular kind. That is not what has been suggested here. Instead, it has been suggested that the kinds of intuitions which make us more appalled by a human being hit on the road than a rabbit, and more appalled by the rabbit than the moth, are grounded in accurate ethical insight into a range of capacities for flourishing between living things.

This reasoning follows very much in the thought of Raimond Gaita to whom this book owes a great debt. In his 'The Philosopher's Dog', Gaita sets forth a compelling case for a common sense, intuitive discrimination between different species and an ethical concern for other animals which does not diminish a primacy of humanity.

> I know of no one whose dog would be treated as equal to a seriously sick infant. If someone did treat their dog like that I would not think of them as a pioneer of ethical thought, but as someone whose sentimentality had made them wicked.
>
> (Gaita 2003, pp. 197–199)

Gaita is not attempting to suggest that *any* need of a human, *any* desire of a human overrides *any* need or *any* desire of a non-human, but what's stopping this?

Since δαίμων comes in degrees, and since humans tend to come somewhere near the highest degree of δαίμων, why, then, doesn't a human demand always override the demand of another living thing?

Since δαίμων is being used here to encompass the broad range of capacities and interests expressed by organisms in general, polio might offer a compelling example of the merits of eradication.[1] None but the terminally macabre would bemoan the eradication of polio. The suffering which this virus brings humanity becomes its primary characteristic; it is 'a disease'.

By shifting the discussion into the realms of the more obviously biological, hordes of parasites raise their ugly heads and still occupy a similarly pathogenic category in our imaginations as that of the viruses. Hundreds of thousands of species on this earth flourish *primarily* by taking away from the flourishing of other species; they feed from, breed within and otherwise totally depend upon the suffering of others.[2] Organisms which have nothing which even resembles a mind, things of short, simple, *almost* automatic existences, lead to terrible suffering in all the other kingdoms of life. The mosquito might have the rudiments of a face, its protrusions echo the limbs of our own ancestors, their flitting and diving speak of the rudiments of desire, but we will justly destroy them, individually and (perhaps) collectively.

Of course, more could be said on the conceptual and ethical differences between the destruction of individual organisms and entire collections of organisms, but the fluidity and breadth of δαίμων can be applied to a collective as easily as it can an individual. The hive flourishes, as does the lone beast. It is this breadth and fluidity (necessary in a discussion of this kind and scale) which makes a broad concept like δαίμων so important. Just as δαίμων is partly defined by the difference in our dismay at a dead moth and a dead badger (or those aspects of that difference corresponding to accurate ethical insight rather than prejudice and mere sentiment) so too does δαίμων encompass the difference between genocide and murder. Scale matters.

So why don't we kill all the wolves and wipe out all the weeds?

Ancient visions of paradise are often of this sort. Milk, honey, no serpents, no diseases.[3] This is the land which was made for me by my ancestors, my green and pleasant land. As I stand in my English country garden, grumbling about foxes and rats, shouldn't I be grateful that I don't need to grumble about wolves and bears also? No poisonous snakes lurk beneath these stones, no scorpions hide in my shoes. Vaccines and antibiotics have rendered most of the more awful diseases a distant cultural memory, problems for distant lands, not my comfy home.

Naïve, arrogant, over-privileged, ethnocentric neo-imperialism! To tell inhabitants of more savage lands that wildlife is in some way precious, that the wolves have a right to existence and that land should be left wild and not cultivated to provide food and wealth for their people. To sit pretty on my green hills and dictate the preservation of the last vestiges of wilderness in the world, what right have I?

As has been a constant theme of this discussion, a dictum by which these theories have been drawn, good philosophy is not about finding absolute and universalisable laws which can be applied to any situation *ad absurdum*, it is about fashioning tools by which the subtle and complex business of life can be best pursued whilst remaining anchored in more lofty principles. Hazy lines drawn in shifting conditions with an eye to a distant light. Ethically orientated compromise is vital.

Athena is not a goddess of warriors, she does not fight with the rage of her brother Ares. Pallas is the quintessence of strategy, she fights with *cleverness*, with circumspection, with compromise.

This discussion began with an exploration of the relationship between σοφία and φρόνησις; it is in the need to negotiate the competing demands encountered in living with other living things that this relationship is both illustrated and employed.

So many times, I have been told by conventional farmers and their sympathisers that urban people just don't understand the reality of living in the country. These townies allow sentiment to overrule what little sense they might have; the cold, hard facts of life in the countryside leave no room for these sorts of delusions. Badgers, foxes, deer, they *need* to be killed so that farmers can make a living, crops *need* to be sprayed, hedgerows and trees *need* to be cut down.

They sit there in their heated tractor cabins, these 'farmers', crushing the life from the soil, they stand in lordly authority over their hundreds of acres and armies of itinerant workers, they collect their vast sums in subsidy and proclaim their rustic wisdom. And it's just too easy.

Bigger harvests, warmer tractors, deadlier poisons, cheaper land, fatter chickens, heavier udders, more pigs per square foot, greater profit... *greater profit.*

Now, I like food, to this my corpulence can testify, nor am I averse to the comforts of technology (similarly evidenced), but when these comforts obscure truths, when ease replaces accuracy, then a fundamental tenet of philosophy has been undermined. The comfort of agribusiness, of industrial-scale witchery, sugar and microwave meals, becomes an extreme which draws humanity away from its true flourishing and into the realms of the unwell. Just as the grand men of Athens were made blind to their true nature by their conventions and ambition, so too do we find ourselves lost. Socrates found the courage to confront these men with the demands of humility, with the discomfort of argumentation, with the need to compromise, and we must similarly compromise.

Of course, Plato's strident attitude has already been described as a problem, and Aristotle's pragmatic circumspection was identified as a possible means of tempering these militant tones, and when it comes to the agrarian concerns of life and death, this temperance can offer the same light as before.

Key to Albert Schweitzer's understanding of the ethical dilemmas involved in treating living things as ends rather than purely as means is an appreciation of the role of *necessity*. There are farmers who have told me that they 'need' to do what they do in order to 'survive'. Do I 'need' to kill the rats?, do I 'need' the eggs which the chickens are laying? Of course, what one means by 'necessity' is determined by the criterion by which that necessity is being judged, a practical value requires practical facts to determine its applicability. Practical necessity (as opposed to logical necessity) is instrumental, X is necessary *for* Y.

Schweitzer's own wrestling with the problem of necessity has been the source of some criticism.[4] On the one hand, Schweitzer identified the prime ethical principle in the requirement to treat all living things as ends in themselves, to respect their will to live, and on the other hand, he acknowledged the inevitability of human life impeding or destroying the lives of other living things (Schweitzer 1923, p. 257). Due to Schweitzer's refusal to acknowledge any explicit hierarchy or differentiation in value between different forms of life (also a source of criticism), the criterion by which necessity could be judged became *biological survival*. As Schweitzer puts it: 'Whenever I injure life of any sort, I must be quite clear whether it is necessary. Beyond the unavoidable, I must never go, not even with what seems insignificant'., p. 264).

Now, it doesn't take a huge leap of the imagination to see that if the criterion for necessity is survival, then a good human life is very swiftly reduced to an ascetic and 'strangely barren' form. Perhaps Schweitzer's own life is testament to an attempt to live such a life of pure service (though we might cruelly characterise his return trips to Gunsbach as hypocrisy), but can we truly recommend that everyone lives as Schweitzer lived? Not only does 'survival' resurrect, once again, the problem of asceticism, but it also raises weird and dreadful thought experiments. As Schweitzer describes in a letter from Lambaréné:

> I always pity the poor fish to the depths of my soul, but I have to choose between killing the fish or the four pelicans who would surely starve to death. I do not know whether I am doing the right thing in deciding one way instead of the other.
>
> (Schweitzer 1951, p. 218)

And what if a crocodile had required Schweitzer's care and the only meat to hand was that of humans? Of course, Schweitzer doesn't mean to suggest that those in danger of death hold absolute ethical preeminence regardless of species, but his difficulty in negotiating the problems of mutually exclusive interests lends weight to the employment of an alternative criterion of necessity.

δαίμων, carrying as it does something of the Hellenistic (or Nussbaumian) notion of 'flourishing', offers an alternative to a purely biological conception of life which enables a more satisfactory negotiation of complex competing demands.

δαίμων does not preclude a life of ascetic service, and there is a certain sense in which they who flourish through a less compromised form of compassion and contemplation may possess greater δαίμων than we who feast and make merry in the blood and sweat of our slaves (but that is a matter for another discussion). δαίμων does, however, permit lives which are good without complete sacrifice and which contain compassion which is full without demanding acts of madness.

When I press my spade into the soil and I know that there is a very good chance I will be destroying lives, hundreds of *minute* lives, this act can be morally laudable. When I spend money on clothes for my daughter and not on veterinary care for an injured mouse, this is not to be condemned. But were I to lace my barn with poison, were I to set about destroying in its entirety the local population of rats in a most painful way and with significant collateral damage, this would not be permissible.

Of course, when normative claims like this are made with little in the way of solid metaethical foundations, rigour is left wanting. *There is nothing in the suggestion* that living things occupy a position on a scale of 'livingness', in part corresponding to our ethical obligations to, and expectations of them, *which tells us just which animals it is and is not all right to kill.*

Schweitzer was left floundering in the ethical conundrums of these many lives, how does δαίμων leave us any flummoxed?

The question stands: why not kill the wolves? Surely they have lesser δαίμων than we, that much seems clear, it takes less to fulfill the potential of a wolf than it does that of most humans. Replace the forests with towns, universities, libraries, even monasteries if you must; the net δαίμων of the world would be increased. How would that world be less philosophical? Certainly, some damage will have been done to achieve this human paradise, but the end result will be increased εὐδαιμονία in its truest form. Or would it? It would certainly have been expedient for Socrates to have lied at his trial, to have used his formidable intellect to outwit his opponents so that he could continue (though perhaps in a truncated form) his educational work. Instead, Socrates decided to look them in the face. Socrates chose not to deal with his enemy in the abstract but instead to confront them and their ideas in their immediate living form. His accusers would have preferred for him to slip away, out of sight, out of mind, to vanish through a cloud of deception, Socrates would not allow them this convenience. Socrates' accusers were forced to get their hands dirty and to look closely upon the damage they were doing. Plato invokes soldierly virtues through his hero and imagines a close bond between these and the other great virtues of which εὐδαιμονία is composed.

Sheer survival might see my garden planted only with potatoes and kale, but I also like beans. Other creatures like beans too and so the business of this little war goes on. But neither side in this conflict bears the other ill will. I find myself just as Schweitzer says 'amidst life which wills to live'. The fact of the matter is just this blunt, this simple, but this simplicity doesn't preclude great lessons in virtue.

On the one hand, what has been said here departs quite markedly from the work of Albert Schweitzer. A significant portion of this discussion has been occupied with the idea that there is a justifiable sense, albeit a complex and relatively vague sense, in which different living things can be treated with more or less ethical concern (or urgency). Schweitzer avoids this differentiation, emphasising instead the common 'will to live' found in all living things. On the other hand, one primary quality of this more nebulous concept of δαίμων, this richness of life, has been not only the extracognitive nature of its composition and extent but also the extracognitive nature of its epistemology. This is to say (and reiterate) that I do not ponder whether or not a pig is a person, nor 'how much' of a person that pig is, I perceive this directly (which is not to say I cannot ponder this personhood, nor that this perception cannot be enriched by more detailed reflections, but only that the basic datum of 'knowing δαίμων', and the virtue of caring about it is primarily visceral not speculative. As Schweitzer says:

> A man is truly ethical only when he obeys the compulsion to help all life that he is able to assist, and shrinks from injuring anything that lives. He does not ask how firmly this or that life deserves one's sympathy as being valuable, nor, beyond that, whether and to what degree it is capable of feeling. Life as such is sacred to him.
>
> (Schweitzer 1923).

Just as I do not deliberate on the personhood of pigs, nor should I think away the 'compulsion to help all life' and shrink 'from injuring anything that lives'. I am justified in feeling greater grief over the suffering of farmed pigs than I do over that of farmed locusts and of exercising great effort in stopping the one and not the other, but this is not the same as feeling *no* grief over the locusts, of feeling *no* compulsion to improve their lot.

We can allow Schweitzer to take us this far at least. Not to a monastery perhaps, but *to guilt*. It may seem odd to say so, but pulling a carrot is not exactly (or solely) a joyous affair. This little life, this thing I have nurtured from seed to full fruit, reaches a point where its death becomes my life. I do not weep for the carrot, there is no gnashing of teeth or rending of garments, but as far as I am able I sustain my sense of death and of a sombre transition.

φρόνησις doesn't give us a route to perfection. The business of φρόνησις is to determine what we are 'able to assist', what the best course of action is, but this does not guarantee we arrive at a situation to celebrate. The right course of action is not necessarily (and perhaps never will be) a truly good course of action.[5]

Schweitzer urges us to keep our ethical activity grounded in an absolute ideal of perfection, that whatever the difficulties of life, however difficult it might be to decide what is best, we must keep a clear view of the goodness by which the whole business is navigated. Virtue in its widest sense, human wisdom, ἀνθρωπίνη σοφία, demands a complex admixture of different virtues, many of which are not cognitive in nature.

Respect (viewed here as synonymous with justice, δικαιοσύνη) courage (ἀνδρεία) and compassion (or charity, or love: ἀγάπη) are, amongst other virtues, vital to εὐδαιμονία. The latter two of these virtues are certainly not of a primarily cognitive nature and the first only partly. φρόνησις alone, with its complex intellectual ways, is not enough (it would just be a collector of facts, details and strategies: a cleverness), it must be part of a complex balance of virtues.

It might seem that an idea like δαίμων twists Schweitzer's vision beyond recognition and is ultimately in direct opposition to it.[6] If one must shrink from injuring anything that lives then how can any hierarchy of 'livingness' correctly inform ethical action? Perhaps when it is built upon (and together with) a variety of insights, including the desire to prevent any harm whatsoever and bring flourishing to all (ἀγάπη). It's not that one virtue, one kind of disposition or way of thinking and feeling, would need to oust the others through some kind of psychological and moral competition, rather they can coexist. Each aspect of the ethical universe paints different aspects of a picture, of a story, and each comes together to form a single, more or less complete understanding of what is right or wrong, *what approximates The Good*, that fulcrum without which no part of the story would have any meaning and by which the whole is judged.

Indeed, in the melting pot of the garden, where the little stories of small lives are played out in such close detail, the virtues, different kinds of ethical disposition and thinking, can be appreciated in their necessarily complex form. An inclination to have every living thing flourishing to its utmost capacity, to see it live long and well, happy and healthy, the desire to keep every creature from pain, every plant from harm, this is a good inclination. This 'reverence for life' is real and deep. This is the foundational virtuous inclination, 'selflessness', with which this discussion began. As has been said, this disposition stretches from how I feel about my daughter to how I feel about my pigs and even my plants. It might be called empathy or love, ἀγάπη or compassion, it doesn't matter too much what we call it, but it is powerful, wonderful and terrible.[7] When I am confronted by images of genocide, of starvation, of dogs having their skin torn from their living bodies, of pigs pushed through steel corridors towards the mechanised jaws of death, buried alive in their thousands, of the quivering body of a poisoned rat, of any countless visions of suffering and death, my blood runs cold and it is as if some essence of my being lurched out to them, my soul tries to save them and cannot.

When ἀγάπη brings us to our knees, when all the world turns to darkness and compassion leaves us lost, φρόνησις picks us up and offers us a short, sharp slap to the face. Enough! All your love is as nothing if you cannot act, if you cannot make some change in your small sphere of influence. These ethical inclinations are not in competition, they are members of a community of ourselves, of our stories, and if thinking of them as homunculi helps us to appreciate the logical and psychological validity of this suggestion, then so be it. But ἀγάπη and φρόνησις get us only so far: to the strangely barren hinterland to which Schweitzer sometimes seems to lead us; this relentless quest for all living things is, although able to compromise, still relatively directionless and prone to lead us into realms of emotional and intellectual inconsistency.

Here is where δικαιοσύνη (respect/justice) steps into the breach. In some ways, justice (the ability to recognise and inclination to act upon what someone deserves) is the result of the interaction of ἀγάπη and φρόνησις. A major aspect of φρόνησις is an ability to differentiate between different kinds of phenomenon, it is an ability to recognise not only the extent of one's own power but also the power of as many other things as possible so that one can determine what can and cannot be achieved and how that might be done; it is the ability to judge consequences. When this inclination to differentiate is combined with an ability to recognise suffering and flourishing and an inclination to increase the latter and decrease the former, justice is a natural mode of resolution.

A sense of justice is not, of course, a purely intellectual thing. As much as protestations of sound legality might claim otherwise, it is not dispassionate. Like φρόνησις, it is manifest in a desire to gain a broad causal view and yet it shares with ἀγάπη an intuitive binding principle.[8] Unlike φρόνησις justice does not seek primarily to distinguish and discover mechanisms, to gain power, instead it drives towards a view of the whole in order to better appreciate how each part fits within that whole under a single principle: something like 'fairness'.

Much of any encounter with δαίμων is achieved through δικαιοσύνη; this is certainly not to claim that perceiving 'livingness' is purely a matter of appreciating what any living thing deserves, only that *a significant part* of this perception is so constituted. But why does this matter? What does this theory of virtues and the pseudo-psychology of moral character have to do with the way in which philosophy as living-with can be practised through permaculture and how to negotiate the competing demands of thousands of non-human organisms?

There are four answers to these questions and they concern: (1) feeling bad (2) courage and honesty, (3) reward and punishment and (4) territory.

Feeling bad

The first and most obvious normative implication of these permaculture virtues is something which has already been stated, namely the way in which negative states should accompany virtuous action: that feeling bad about doing the best thing is entirely appropriate.

'Feeling bad' is not entirely synonymous with guilt. Guilt conveys a quite one-dimensional kind of regret and neglects other ethically important kinds of attitude.

Confusion about the meaning of regret isn't a preserve of academic speculation. A common example of when people become confused about the appropriateness of 'feeling bad' is when people say 'I'm sorry' upon hearing about another's misfortune. This confusion may be more prevalent amongst the British, with their penchant for saying 'sorry' about almost anything, but many of us will be familiar with the way this kind of 'apology' is dismissed as inappropriate. Perhaps one person will have experienced an inconvenience, maybe bad traffic, and another will respond: 'I'm sorry' to which the first will answer: 'why? It's not your fault.' Now, this is to confuse two senses of 'I'm sorry'. One sense of 'I'm sorry' is something like: 'I regret that *I made* this (or allowed this to) happen' (with an implicit recognition that one will attempt to ensure that it doesn't happen again). Another sense of 'I'm sorry' is more like: 'I regret that this happened' or 'I wish that this thing had not happened', without any recognition of personal responsibility. This latter apology is meant as a condolence and an attempt to express solidarity (*'you're not alone in your pain, I'm here with you'*). Indeed, this latter kind of apology can be quite general and take the form of 'I wish the world were not the sort of place that this kind of thing happens', recognising that we are all, whether currently suffering or not, in the same leaky boat.

This distinction between guilt (personally responsible regret) and condolence (general regret) is crucial to understanding the appropriate bad feeling when confronted with negotiating competing demands between living things. This distinction is crucial, however, not because it exhausts the possibilities for an appropriate bad feeling, but because it does not.

It might seem straightforward to categorise appropriate bad feelings when doing what seems best as belonging to the second (condolence) form of bad feeling, but this doesn't make for a good fit. When I am letting my dogs run amok in the barns in the hope that they will scare away the rats, and when they catch and kill a rat, my role in that death is clear. When I stand over the little corpse of that rat and say sorry, my apology is not simply an expression of general regret at the state of our broken world, it is something *more personal* and, simultaneously, *less regretful*.

If one were to be speaking to a survivor of some calamity, a really dreadful injustice (perhaps a natural disaster or genocide) in which innocent people were hurt and killed, the sense in which one would express regret, 'I'm so sorry', would be entirely non-responsible and entirely heartfelt. In a quite powerful and clear way, one would wish that those things simply had not happened. When one is confronted with all the little acts of destruction, bloody or otherwise, which are part of permaculture, one is intimately aware not only of one's own responsibility in these acts but also of how both these acts and the scenarios which make them necessary are *not entirely regrettable*.

Now, the tension involved in an idea of incomplete regret, with its psychological, ethical and logical peculiarities, will be explored more fully in the close of this discussion; what is crucial here is to recognise that there are forms of feeling bad which do not directly entail a desire for the situation to be otherwise. This lack of regret is, in a fairly obvious sense, a consequence of doing the right thing, of acting in a way which seems, both prior to and after the event, to have been the correct and morally laudable way of acting. In this way, it is possible to imagine a situation in which one's own personal responsibility has resulted in a better state of affairs despite the overall state of affairs remaining, in some sense, upsetting. So, in this way, the death of the rats is less bad than my family not having access to organic eggs. I know that if I were to buy eggs from the shop, these eggs will have involved far more processing and logistical complexity. A broad and detailed assessment of the mechanisms involved in getting any item of food permits me to understand the amount of labour, suffering and death necessary to achieve sustenance within a geographically diffuse and economically specialised system. Quite apart from concerns about fuel, space, workers' rights, hen welfare, antibiotic resistance, chemical leaching, water expenditure, corruption, supermarket monopolies or a thousand other things, rats will still have been killed to get these other eggs, it's just that someone else will have done the killing.

One of the most obvious and more naïve responses to this recognition of the suffering involved in consumption is to consume as little as possible. Of course, this line of reasoning needn't be so short-sighted as to fail to see the ascetic extremities to which it might lead if left in its most uncompromising, ad absurdum form, that would be an uncharitable formulation of such an objection. If the game being played is 'where do I draw the line?' then it is easy enough to imagine someone who suggests the line should be drawn elsewhere (in whichever direction and however marginally). 'Give up eggs, but not courgettes'. This is certainly somewhere that calculations and intuitions of justice start to be important, but it is important to first understand what might drive us to draw the line more or less in one direction or another: consume less or consume more? Is it 'feeling bad' which we are trying to avoid? Is there a line which can be drawn by which we might finally breathe a sigh of relief, having shed the dreadful responsibility for suffering; a point at which we can exit these stories of death? This certainly seems to be a significant source of motivation for both those who feel justified in placing great importance on human needs and those who place great importance on the suffering of non-human organisms.

And yet, this escape from feeling bad is less pronounced amongst permaculturists and homesteaders. I have had plenty of conversations with people who have found their comfortable niche in the world of consumption: vegans and carnists alike. So many people have firm ideas about what matters and what doesn't and how they can ensure they are able to entirely avoid doing morally relevant harm: shorn of responsibility. Not real permaculturists though.

Certainly, there is a spectrum of ethical insight amongst all groups and it has never been an aim of this discussion to suggest that there is any guaranteed way of attaining such insight, but a lack of comprehensive certainty is not the same as a lack of educational excellence. A method of education can be good, even best, without being perfect. Nor has it been the purpose of this discussion to ascertain the degree to which the correlation between permaculture and ethical insight is causal, that would be an empirical study of a quite different character (though a study worth pursuing). No, this is (amongst other things) a qualitative treatment of my own life with permaculture. One person's account of their own experience of an educational experience can be as valuable in informing a broader view of the value of that experience as any statistical analysis of many such individuals. I can say without hesitation that life lived in close proximity with other living things, from them and with them, *can be* ethically informative. This educational relationship is (amongst other more complex relationships) causal. And part of this life lived with other living things is talking to other permaculturists.

I can talk philosophy almost inexhaustibly: ad nauseam. It infuriates and galls those who do not share this disposition. I can shift in and out of political and metaphysical speculation with relative ease and, crucially, relish. I find 'small talk' quite difficult and I am inclined to attempt to push the conversation in the direction of abstract and ethical debate. I suspect this gadflyish talk is part of the Socratic dream. There are perhaps a few other subjects on which I can pontificate with similar zeal, perhaps, but none come even close to matching permaculture-talk. Permaculture-talk and philosophy-talk vie for the top spot, and permaculture-talk is often more sociable.

Not long ago, I was doing a bit of voluntary pottering in a garden at a multi-faith ashram in West Wales. Over my years of visiting the ashram, I have become friends with the monk responsible for the vegetable garden. At first, it was simply a matter of volunteering for a task in which I had some skill (and some enthusiasm) but it takes mere moments for two permaculturists to get into permaculture-talk; and permaculture-talk is sudden, swift, deep and familiar. So, the monk and I would talk about this weed or that, the way this soil behaves or how elephant poo compares with horse poo. Weather-talk (which might otherwise fit firmly into the 'small talk' category) takes on a new and powerful dimension in the realm of permaculture. Each shift in the season, every shower and every dry spell is reflected in the performance of each different kind of vegetable. Cold winters can lead to good fruit, dry springs can lead to dead seedlings and late plantings. But very few permaculturists grow exactly the same vegetables as one another, different tastes, soils and climates mean different crops and so we may find the year's weather has treated one of us kindly and the other cruelly. And all this talk somehow feels like it is happening as a small instance, fleeting and fragile, amongst a truly vast and ancient tradition of small scale self-provision. Thousands, indeed tens of thousands of years and miles and acres and billions, trillions of conversations all about similar things. And it happens during work, it happens as you scrape your hands through rock and soil, as you heave at roots and gently place seedlings into new ground.

On one occasion, without any introduction or even a moment's silence, I found myself planting out chard with another volunteer, a regular, and we got to talking about toads. We both like toads. She was interested to learn that toads are, along with Ravens and humans, the longest living land animal of these islands. I was interested to learn where and how she has encountered toads in the sides of beds. But we also talked about killing things.

When one sows seed (always depending upon the species of vegetable) it is common to sow more than is needed. This is a sensible course of action since many may die, they might be eaten by slugs or snails, mice or voles, and some of them may just fail to germinate. So, to ensure that you have enough seedlings it is wise, it is prudent, to sow more than needed. But this often leaves unwanted plants. Now, many people will exchange extra seedlings and the trade between permaculturists is one of the greatest joys of the business. I will never come home from the ashram without some new vegetable in seed or seedling form. But this is often not possible and quite apart from this, it is also wise to plant only the strongest seedlings. Of all the plants which do germinate and of those which survive, many are simply inferior. 'A proper gardener' she called me when I showed almost no concern over thinning (killing off the weaker plants). She felt bad about it, she wanted to give them all a life if she could, to find a place for them. Of course, this might sound like sentimental rubbish which would be un unsurprising find in a volunteer at an ashram, but actually, it was said with a level head and no hyperbole. 'A proper gardener'; I'm not sure about that, I think perhaps I can be guilty of forgetting about the destruction I am causing: desensitised. This volunteer's reluctance to kill the weak plants was a healthy reminder, it wasn't a move away from the reality of the situation, not some fantastical metaphysical trip into a realm of crystals and angelic healing, no, it was a move closer, a simple shift in attention towards the life in my hands. I killed them still and felt worse about it. We both felt a little bit bad about it and carried on.

I have only been deer stalking once, only once with the aim of hunting deer and killing them and I was not the shooter. There were no deer shot that day, but we did skin a deer which was shot previously. I have met many people who shoot deer triumphantly but there was no chance I would go hunting with one of those people, I have never been so unfortunate as to think that would be a good idea. No, the hunter with whom I skinned the deer handled the dead animal with respect. Revulsion was certainly not part of the picture but a quiet and constant understanding of the deer in life as well as in death was in the air. Permaculture can be as simple as this. It needn't be a wholesale revision of lifestyle in order to qualify, it can be partial, it can be gradual, but it must take Schweitzer's principle of a reverence for life, of a far-reaching compassion, and apply this through an ever greater closeness with that life: proximal, practical, intellectual and emotional closeness. Killing a deer, a creature so full of life, of desires, joys and pains, certainly represents an act of significant destruction: a dramatic act against the interests of a living thing, a person, a δαίμων, and yet, when it is committed with a keen sense of the loss involved, with a bad feeling, and with a sophisticated recognition of (and motivation against) the complex systems of suffering and degradation which have been avoided through this act of killing, then it cannot *so easily* be seen as contrary to a reverence for life. And this happens, when the destruction of life is approached with compassion, prudence and *honesty*, darkness is preserved. I have seen it in hunters and permaculturists (sometimes they are the same), in those who will themselves closer into the source of things, into the beating heart of the systems upon which their own existence must depend and refuse to close themselves off from the pain.

This 'bad feeling' doesn't require regret. Certainly, in form this bad feeling does resemble the second kind of regret identified above, but what is most crucial to this resemblance is not regret but, rather, *solidarity*. With the first form of regret it shares a recognition of personal responsibility (though in this instance for an act designed to be morally laudable) and it combines this sense of causal responsibility with a recognition of the inherent value of that which has been infringed upon. To recognise other living things as ends in themselves is to recognise the responsibility to share in their pain, to be present with that pain, with their loss (however small and trivial that loss may seem).

Of course, I am not attempting to recommend that we should be breaking down in tears each time we pull a carrot out of the ground, the extent of the 'bad feeling' must follow a sense of δαίμων and of justice: a tear for a carrot would be silly but for a pig, it would not. What is crucial is that our motivation is not an escape from a responsibility for suffering, indeed it is almost the opposite. Our motivation can be mixed, it must be mixed in the sense of different virtuous dispositions interacting in complex ways (often in complementary as opposed to competitive ways), but when a desire to eliminate suffering (compassion) is combined with a desire to flourish individually (and tribally or familially) one can and should arrive at a sense of the need to share in the suffering one has caused. This need is driven not only by a desire to appreciate in the fullest sense the truth of what one is engaged in (honesty/curiosity) it is also driven by a desire that each thing receives that it deserves (justice) and a more general desire for fellowship, or communion.

This is the 'thick' nature of symbiotic ethics; stories play out in complex ways, but this need not translate into ethical aporia, rather it means that familiar ethical precepts and virtues need to accommodate one another in subtle ways which reflect the reality of lived experience. Certainly, one could attempt to offer very specific normative instructions on the basis of this kind of ethical reflection. One might, for example, suggest that it is never justifiable to kill pigs in order to eat them since pigs are just too much persons, too much δαίμων, too much to lose. In support of such a suggestion, one might offer accounts of interactions with pigs, stories of our lives together. Indeed, there was one particular occasion on which I was brought to tears by living with pigs.

I was fencing off a new area for the pigs, an area of thick brush and hedge which I had planned to make into a lawn for my daughter. The pigs are very good at clearing this sort of growth and it would both save me the effort and give them something nice to eat and interesting to do. At the entrance to this new run was an area which I had previously been used to burn various old waste, organic and otherwise. The two larger, older pigs had very little trouble in ignoring this patch of burnt ground but the two smaller pigs were less keen. These two just loitered on the near side of the burn area and sniffed the edges gingerly. When they become cautious like this, they begin to make quiet noises, grunts and squeals under their breath, back and forth they make these noises as they shift their feet tentatively.

I attempted to coax these two pigs into leaping the bonfire site. I used an old pallet as a pig-board and gradually decreased their space until there was really only one direction in which to go. The male, Button Mushroom, finally plucked up the courage and joined the big pigs in their lush, new ground, but the little girl, Squash, she stayed behind. I'm not sure how long we were there, me pushing her gently towards the scorched soil, her pushing back and growling in barely audible discontent. A long while. She crawled up a steep bank at the side rather than move onto the ash and bit by bit she became introverted and visibly frightened. In the end, I abandoned the pig-board and crouched beside her. She has such pretty eyes, framed by tortoiseshell lashes, but they were distant and lonely now, and beneath her thick skin, I could feel tremors in the tension of her body. Each breath came out with desperate little cries. So, I held her and talked gently about nothing in particular. It was a long while. Pigs smell like white pepper and they are full of self.

My thoughts drifted to all those other pigs. Philosophy bids us look to the whole, to find detail in the present but not to be confined by it, to discover the meaning, the significance of that detail by discovering its wider context. So out there, beyond this little trial, were millions of pigs in steel boxes, millions of eyes like these being thrown onto conveyer belts and crushed into machines of death. Broken bones, screaming, confusion, air thick with fear. I have seen the videos, seen the malpractice, seen the 'good practice'. So, I held her closer, and I talked more gently, and I wept.

She walked across the ashes eventually, with tears on her back.

But no attempt is being made at such specific normative instructions. Perhaps somewhere, at some time, under certain circumstances, it has been right to kill and eat a pig, I have insufficient powers of φρόνησις to scry such distant, absolute details. Such knowledge, such grand, absolute moral truths, is the wisdom of Apollo, not of humans. In my garden, alongside my pigs, I find the possibility of eating a pig being justifiable barely comprehensible, just as I find scenarios in which eating humans can be justified equally incomprehensible. But there are many gardens in the world, many stories. No, following the work of Albert Schweitzer, the suggestion here is that the most crucial work of philosophy (in its written and most theoretical form) is to help shape our motivations, to offer new ways of understanding what should inform our decisions and actions, not (at least in the first instance) to speculate about particular kinds of decisions and actions. So, feeling bad about X or Y is not as important as recognising that it is often right to feel bad even when doing the right thing. By taking familiar and widely accepted virtues as axioms and then placing them in the context of living with other living things, it is suggested that new and more complete systems of moral learning can be illuminated. In the end, it helps you to be more careful.

In its most basic form the suggestion is that life lived with other living things can help to illustrate that:

- The basic desire for all living things to flourish is ineliminable from, though not necessarily sovereign over (necessary but not sufficient for) right moral deliberation and action. This desire for universal flourishing is concomitant with a desire to limit suffering as far as possible.
- Not only are death and suffering inevitable but human flourishing will necessarily entail the suffering and death of other living things.
- A recognition that not all flourishing and suffering is of equivalent moral weight should not lead to a negation of the desire for *all* living things to flourish. Nor should the desire for *all* living things to flourish lead to a diminishment of a desire for personal flourishing. Despite prima facie encounters with these problems, these various dispositions are commensurate (these dispositions can and should survive this conflict).
- Other virtuous dispositions can assist in negotiating this apparent conflict, one of which (closely related to both compassion and honesty) is a desire to share in the lives (joys and pains) of others, and particularly those for whom we bear more direct responsibility. This solidarity in suffering is crucial to overall virtue (wisdom).

I have known farmers who feel bad and I have known farmers who do not, the former are, without exception, better people.

'Feeling bad' is, of course, a quite two-dimensional sort of phrase. I have no doubt that even those farmers who suggest that the suffering of their animals is not morally relevant do, in some respects, 'feel bad' about this suffering. Quite probably the only kind of human which could escape any kind of 'feeling bad' in the face of suffering would not really be a human at all, they would be lacking something central; we would probably call them a psychopath and indeed their δαίμων would be very unwell. But the key to the idea of 'feeling bad' being discussed here is the way in which it is embraced. This 'feeling bad' is not to be regretted, avoided, denied or dissimulated in any way. This is a feeling bad which is parallel to and compatible with 'feeling good'.

Indeed, when I slice through the writhing length of an earthworm as I dig in my vegetable beds, not only should I attend to that mangled thing and dwell (if only for slightly longer than a fleeting moment) in the darkness I have brought into that little world, I should feel joy in the vegetables themselves and in my act of producing food (which will taste nice and be nutritious) for myself and my family. Just as the dispositions which give rise to these feelings of sadness and joy can and should cohabit our souls, so too should the feelings themselves cohabit.[9]

Within the permaculture garden itself, within the wild world of living things, there is a model of this cohabitation. Conflict is not illusory and yet a healthy and sustainable system, a biome which can flourish in stable persistence ad infinitum, depends upon a complex admixture of seemingly antagonistic forces which, due to subtle mechanisms and distinct approaches, coexist and constitute vital components of the thriving whole. This is a lesson of permaculture: we are *identical* with the biome... but more on this later.

Solidarity is not the only necessary virtue.

Courage and honesty

So far, this negotiation of difficult situations and the avoidance of vice through the balancing of various dispositions may sound quite strongly Aristotelean, but it is with Plato's soldierly virtues that the most stark lessons of permaculture are learned (Plato, *Apol.*, 28ᵃ–29ᵇ).

Honesty denies us the ease of looking away, of ignoring the pain, and combined with a desire for flourishing in ourselves and all living things, it can bring us to a lesson of solidarity and sadness, to the sharing of pain. But sadness, 'feeling bad', can be debilitating. This reaching out to those around us and taking responsibility for our actions is a very local pursuit. This is not to claim that the solidarity which has been outlined is a purely passive thing, such unflinching contact can take enormous effort, but understanding the compatibility of 'feeling bad' and doing the right thing, is not the same as understanding the strength necessary to achieve this effort of communion, nor the ethical and intellectual context in which it is appropriate (what are the broader implications of this feeling bad? What impact does this appropriate negativity have on our wider ethical conduct?).

It is easy enough to conceive of what is meant by 'honesty' here. Looking into the eyes of a cockerel as you slice off his head and feeling the desperate convulsions of his body, the warmth of his blood, these are the brutal and direct facts of killing. Lived-honesty is not a very far cry from intellectual honesty. When I have a metaphysical opinion, I have an intellectual duty to become familiar with the various facts and arguments upon which that position rests. When I am going to benefit from some food, I have a similar (if not ethically identical) responsibility to become intimately familiar with the processes by which this food becomes available to me.

It might be suggested that practical honesty and theoretical honesty are ethically distinct insofar as familiarity with the theoretical under-pinnings of a metaphysical position can be achieved without a complete alteration of lifestyle and that one can be theoretically familiar with the practical reality without being practically familiar with the processes. Knowing how a chicken gets on to the plate doesn't necessitate putting it there personally.

This sort of objection would: (1) reflect a lack of appreciation of the kind of wealth and leisure necessary to devote time to metaphysical speculation (and would therefore almost certainly come from someone who enjoyed those benefits) and (2) fail to appreciate the analogous way in which meta-physical positions and their arguments can be learned by rote without gen-uine understanding and that in order for a theoretical position to be truly understood in the way that it should be, the arguments and facts upon which it depends should be fully *understood* each time the position is expressed or made use of. So, it wouldn't even be enough to have killed a chicken once upon a time and to thus express a true understanding of the processes lead-ing to the chicken dinner, this would leave the rest of the occasions crucially wanting.

Of course, when dealing with persons, with living things (with δαίμων), there is the added (and ethically more urgent) quality of needing to deal with the living things involved as ends in themselves as opposed to means to an end. Arguments upon which an opinion rests do not share this same vital quality. Certainly, when one is communicating a metaphysical position part of the impetus for communicating that position truthfully and rigorously is out of respect for the person with whom one is communicating (whether that person be oneself or otherwise). In this way, these two forms of honesty do mirror one another since even abstract, argumentative honesty is aimed at treating persons as ends in themselves.[10] The added ethical urgency in the case of practical honesty comes from the closer relationship between ends and means: it is frequently 'necessary' to treat persons (δαίμων) as means as well as ends and the danger of treating them *solely* as means is more imme-diately present.[11]

I once said to a group of friends that I thought people who were not some kind of vegetarian were necessarily stupid, lazy or evil (the group was not solely or even largely composed of confessed vegetarians). There was cer-tainly a sense in which I wished to be provocative (the provocation largely worked) but I could also now comfortably amend this initial proposition to the suggestion that people who are not some form of *vegan* are stupid, lazy or evil.

This amendment may seem unimportant and this anecdote certainly does not represent a clumsy effort to veer off into the specifics of vegan vs vegetarian ethics (a boggy area of ethical debate at the best of times), no, the point is that *I am often not some form of vegan*. I claimed above that I don't buy eggs or dairy products because this was a step too far, but it would not be true to say that I *never* go too far: sometimes I do and, when I do, it is because I am *lazy*. Perhaps Peter Singer is right that there are times when not being vegan is strategically sound for the sake of not scaring carnivores away from the idea of vegetarianism (Singer 2006), and his idea that the occasional luxury is justifiable is entirely commensurate with the model of flourishing (and a non-ascetic ethic) which has been expressed here.[12] But there are times when the luxury is not justified, when I know what suffering lead to this palm oil or that avocado, and I just plug up the ears of my conscience and indulge. In fact, one way or another, I do this all the time.

'Stupid' is very different from 'lazy' and 'evil' is barely interesting at all. 'Stupid' is just an abrasive way of saying 'ignorant', which is to indicate those people who haven't had access to the lessons of permaculture or philosophy (who haven't been properly exposed to the way in which living things should be treated as ends in themselves), they just don't know about δαίμων. 'Evil' would just be something like the 'psychopath' mentioned above, someone who is so broken that they just don't feel any compassion at all. No, 'lazy' has something to do with a lack of strength and a willing suspension of virtues. I can see that a bowl of chips would do very nicely, hardly a mortification, but I begin to shut down the extent of my vision, my φρόνησις, I narrow my focus to mere words on the menu and the smells in the kitchen so that options begin to seem equivalent.

I do this because it's easier. Feeling simultaneously bad and good about an action which has obviously negative impacts but is nonetheless laudable is entirely possible in a temporally, geographically and causally limited frame of reference, but when φρόνησις brings to the fore an entire world of inexorably linked causes and consequences, the chain of death and suffering can seem overwhelming. It can be very tempting to shut down φρόνησις almost entirely. What's needed is *courage* and *honesty*.

The aim of my provocation was to frame that discussion of animal ethics away from compassion, and the criticisms of 'mere sentiment' which that kind of motivation can engender. There are obviously occasions when a passionate investment of care coupled with a lack of critical rigour, of hard-headed φρόνησις, can justifiably be called sentimental in a bad sense. The recognition of, say, suffering or pain in another animal can cause a kind of sympathetic shock and result in an inclination to overstretch the importance of an event or imbue some behaviour with qualities which are not extant. This is what might be called 'mere sentiment', since, as Gaita explains, there are clearly times when the recognition of important emotional states through these kinds of compassionate sympathies are perfectly accurate and not at all 'mawkish or sentimental' (Gaita 2003, p. 115). I had hoped that by reaching beyond compassion into the realms of virtues less prone to wayward accusations of effeminate inaccuracy, I might hope to set a spark in regions of souls otherwise untouched by the motivation of compassion.

Courage and honesty (ἀνδρεία and ἀλήθεια) inhabit a different (though, crucially, not unconnected) section of our souls from compassion/charity/universal love. These are very active virtues, fiery things. I suspect that diligence occupies a similarly active region. So, calling people lazy, weak, cowardly, pathetic hits a somewhat different nerve from that exercised by charges of cruelty, unfeeling disregard and callousness. People can, at least in certain cultures, become proud of their callouses far easier than they can their indolence or cowardice.

Not to be a vegan, then, is to indulge in languid lethargy; unwilling to embrace their moral responsibilities, these pathetic people (we) would rather hide behind screens of self-deception and divided labour than face the truth! We, wretches all, might construct clever little arguments to defend our comfort, no doubt we have the luxury of time and wealth that we might collude in such sophistry, but seen in the cold light of the real world, thrown down into the filth and blood upon which our delicate intellectual ornaments rest, these constructions unravel with merciless speed.

Perhaps this is the sort of militant diatribe which Singer imagines scaring away the carnists.

But we are all lazy, some more than others, we constantly find ourselves at something resembling the infinitesimal juncture of volition and compulsion, of responsibility and disease which was outlined at the outset of this discussion. A lack of courage or honesty can feel like a condition over which one has no control, how can one hope to 'create' the power to gain power over oneself? Yet underneath this despair there lurks that aching nausea of personal responsibility, that nagging presence of one's own agency. But this kind of existential or solipsistic reflection is a fantasy of which, as we have seen, Aristotle is keenly aware, our agency is a thing 'amidst'. Whether I can muster the courage to take action, to tell the truth, is linked closely to the stories unfolding about me, of that which is present to me. We can take measures to ensure our environments encourage virtue, φρόνησις can assist ἀνδρεία: when all is well in the cosmos Athena is allied to Ares. The general who hides miles from the front, in cushioned comfort and safety, spends lives as if they were a pittance. Permaculture, in its small way, is an effort to step forward into the fray, to view the battle in its bloody reality.

The combination of ἀγάπη and φρόνησις, and of a recognition of the validity and ethical necessity of sadness, can threaten a kind of unsustainable spiral into despair. As I held that little pig and thought of all those millions of pigs, past, present and future, the darkness loomed. What permaculture represents is a means of training, of strengthening; the only way to combine these apparently overwhelming moral inclinations in an emotionally sustainable way is to find a way through the darkness, to find a way not to turn back but to forge ahead to the unified, balanced virtue on the other side, to σοφία.

When Odysseus knew that he must sail past the sirens to reach his destination he would not close his own ears to their song, that would have been dishonest, it would have undermined his entire way of being, it would have made the destination meaningless; what is the return of a master if he is not worthy of being a master? Instead, Athena's champion lashed himself to his mast, he threw himself into certain torment with the solid assurance of his vessel and crew as both a means of progress and a guarantee against self-destruction. Odysseus' courage without cleverness would have been worthless: deadly; his cleverness without courage would have been impotent and speculative; without the drive to hear the truth of the siren song and without the strength of bravery to undergo that voyage he would have been just another lost Argive. Athena's champion had both courage and cleverness.

Permaculture is just such a vessel. This might seem somewhat of a melodramatic appraisal of a simple, genteel, pastoral occupation, but it is a method for confronting ourselves with the truth of the means upon which our existence depends whilst doing so in an emotionally and psychologically sustainable way.

The truth of our lives, the world upon which we depend, is not a causally narrow thing. Temporally and geographically, our lives are part of a vast and sprawling universe teaming with ethically relevant events. So, permaculture might be deemed a petty gesture. There are sweatshops and concentration camps, genocides and slavery, gargantuan machines of imperial and market consumption. The horror of Leviathan; the horror! What is this spec of dirt in this maelstrom of life and death? Well, perhaps its smallness is important, and perhaps its smallness is deceptive.

As has been said, the context of our lives is not temporally narrow, we are not just what we are right now. The stories of our lives may indeed feature a central character (or characters) as Ricoeur suggests, but whether we are author or reader it would be a mistake to concentrate on this slim volume at the centre.[13] The philosopher is a student of the epics of life which reach out in every direction: a spherical library suffused with themes. And look! In each volume there is a hand in the soil, a hand young and full, a hand old and weathered, a hand grasping leaves and roots, wiping a tired brow, catching rain, wielding a well-worn tool, shooing away the beaks and claws, caressing a snout and a bristly back, wiping away the blood, feeding the mouth young and full, feeding the mouth old and weathered. Here's that hand, and here again.

The power of becoming that hand should not be underestimated. The power of embodying that kind of historically extended self can be as ethically informative as all the learned treatises of the world combined. In permaculture is a vessel with a deaf crew which can take me into an awareness of this extended self. I could throw myself into the front lines, into the desperate subjugation of the diamond mine or the stinking gore of the killing floor; then the sirens could scream their song at full and terrible volume; but what then? Perhaps there is a time and place to stand at the front of the battle, to push into the fiery heat of raw destruction, but who could withstand such a blaze for more than a moment? Ares alone can fight so ceaselessly; Athena is our goddess and she picks her moments.

So, permaculture thrusts us into smaller darknesses, to blisters, and blood, and filth, and freezing rain, but it also offers us a deaf and steady crew, and a mast to which we might bind ourselves. Nowhere to run now, king of Ithaca! Cleverest of all the Achaeans! Neither flight nor self-destruction is yours to choose. Witness the turning of the world! Feel the pain of labour, the aching cost; weigh the preciousness of the food you eat!

This kind of ethic, of the importance of bringing oneself closer to the source of one's flourishing, of having enough courage and honesty to do so, has much in common with political philosophies of alienation and that similarity should be acknowledged. Even in its more traditional socioeconomic sphere, this concept of separation needn't be confined to motivations for profit or a distancing from our own nature, as Sanderson and Pugliese suggest:

> Marx described other forms of alienation that he believed capitalism produces. Instead of valuing workers as human beings who are ends in themselves, the capitalist treats workers as means to the end of profit.
>
> (Sanderson and Pugliese 2012, p. 253)

It is, once again, Kant's second formulation which lies at the heart of this separation. Schweitzer's reformulation of this central ethical principle to include all living things hinges (in part) on an idea of our own inextricable place within this ethical whole: 'I am life which wills to live, and I exist *in the midst of* life which wills to live'. It is this 'amidstness' which permaculture can bring to the fore.

The particular kind of amidstness, of dealienation, which permaculture can instill is as broad as the concept itself[14]:

1   *Social Dealienation*: An awareness of the labour and suffering (human and otherwise) behind the things we consume and active participation in taking direct responsibility for that labour and suffering.
2   *Environmental and Economic Dealienation*: A direct encounter with the materials of upon which our flourishing depends, on the full nature and preciousness of our food and of the complex interconnection of living systems and our biological and ethical role in them.
3   *Personal Dealienation*: The process of becoming directly familiar with δαίμων, allowing oneself to be exposed to and to 'see' the personness and purposiveness of other living things (accurate sentiment as opposed to 'mere sentiment').

4 *Seasonal (or 'cosmic') Dealienation*: A keen sense of the non-biological components of the living system, a direct and highly aesthetic sense of the scale and majesty of life on earth. (A less obviously ethical kind of dealienation but a crucial part of the lesson in wisdom and wellbeing which permaculture offers and which will be elaborated on below).

One reason this similarity with alienation is important is that it can act as a theoretical shortcut to the ethical expansiveness of this theory of symbiotic ethics through permaculture.

Having asserted the continuity of ethical relevance between living things (whilst not wholly endorsing the ethical equivalence sometimes suggested by Schweitzer) the reality of conflict and an intuitive prioritisation of humanity (or at least moral relevance of δαίμων) leaves this vague ethic of 'livingness' decidedly wanting in normative, instructional potency. To those who find domination attractive, in those souls where compassion finds less comprehensive purchase, the topography of conduct must highlight new features.

The socio-political axioms which inform modern ethical debate have secured a familiar way of talking about the ethics of economics. To ask why I should pay attention to the working conditions of those who make my clothes, to ask why it is important to regard humans on the other side of the globe as persons like myself (in ethically relevant ways) is, in certain respects, fatuous. Whatever empathy may or may not be at play, a closing of the gap, a willingness and desire to see the reality is a core principle of justice. Broad and entrenched ideas of honesty and courage do inform our understanding of what might be called honourable conduct, of treating people as they should be treated: not only as means but also as ends. Taking our earplugs out (or never putting them in) is not a remotely novel ethic, putting this kind of idea into practice is far more challenging than grasping the validity of the motivation.

Finding the right environment suited to opening our abilities of accurate, ethical perception is crucial to (or even largely constitutive of) effective and sound ethical learning. This is a more subtle and complex business than these epistemic platitudes might suggest. Sometimes what seems to be a close familiarity can exacerbate inaccurate prejudices as much as, if not more than vast distances and disengagement. Neighbourhoods seething with racial hatred can have their preconceptions compounded through personal experience, flames which are only fanned by a distant and liberal class of lawmakers who can seem so ignorant of lived realities. Farmers who see their animals every day allow anonymity, numbers and a culture of strength, pragmatism and the necessity of callousness to shape their 'realism'. Permaculture is not only a vessel through the Siren song of our less admirable inclinations, it also charts a more subtle course along a knife-edge between distance and contact, between Scylla and Charybdis, between bloody conflict and ignorant oblivion.

Permaculture has been intentionally shaped in a holistic way to be a method of confronting social and environmental problems in the widest possible way. By growing our own food (in however marginal or complete a way) we familiarise ourselves with processes which involve non-humans *and* humans throughout the world. The rain my plants need teaches me about those who suffer drought and those who are washed away by floods and all the while maintaining a keen sense of the beauty of the water itself. Loosing cabbages to caterpillars may not endanger the lives of my family but it helps me understand those who do live in such peril. And all the while I can keep sight of the butterflies as butterflies; those who merely walk in the hills and marvel at these splendid insects, their vibrant colours and elegant flight, risk abandoning themselves to vapid, contemplative removal, to Charybdis' watery ignorance.

Of course, permaculture represents more than just a method of self-help, of neo-hellenistic self-cultivation. By growing my own cabbage that is one cabbage I don't need to buy, it is one less thing which will add to the vast and spiralling mechanism of industrial agriculture and market consumption. In a tangible and immediately apparent way, there is a causal relationship between living this 'good life' and taking a personal role in social and environmental justice (albeit largely through refusing to take part in bad rather than actively preventing it). This activity thus affords an unusually palpable species of a consequentialist lesson.

This kind of utilitarian impact of small-scale sustainable self-provision might seem a striking omission from what has been discussed so far in relation to the ethical value of permaculture. This avoidance has, however, been for three principal reasons: First, the more practical merits of this kind of lifestyle are complex and their sheer multiplicity would require an entire book to do them anything approaching justice (tempting but also widely attempted elsewhere).[15] Secondly, the measurable impact of such a lifestyle requires not only empirical evidence but is also highly contestable. Thirdly, before any systematic treatment of the practical merits of permaculture could be attempted, it would first be necessary (or appropriate) to gain a firm and plausible understanding of the kind of metaethics upon which any such merit was based.

Before we can say that permaculture is good because soil bacteria, physical activity, sunlight and organic vegetable-based diets have been shown to combat, say, depression, we would need to know far more about what we mean by 'depression' and why it is something we should avoid. Before we attempt to discuss the way in which growing our own beans can help us boycott corrupt farming industries which prop-up slavery and violent juntas, we need to know how we should think about our own roles in a global economy and the nature of our responsibilities to such distant people. Before we can properly talk about all the different ways in which we can withdraw support from industrial animal farming and prevent the suffering of non-humans, we need to have a better appreciation of why we would even bother trying that in the first place. Indeed, this has been one of the ways in which this discussion has sought to emulate the work of Albert Schweitzer: by taking absolutely fundamental principles of philosophy as the necessary starting point of any ethical discussion and attempting to suggest that besides the laudable practical impacts of permaculture, the experience and actives of permaculture can play a pivotal role in informing how we approach much more general kinds of questions (questions which are logically prior to any more practical discussion).

Whilst this kind of logical supersession does play a significant role in the shape of this discussion it is also important to note that many of the ethical lessons of permaculture discussed so far would be fairly vacuous without the assumption that some kind of practical impact was being made through the activities taking place. If growing a cabbage obviously doesn't help anyone, if keeping pigs leads to more harm than good, if sifting soil were demonstrably detrimental to one's health and an act of relentless drudgery then the 'moral growth' discussed so far would be a hollow if not contradictory achievement. It would be a purely ascetic self-flagellation of the kind dismissed at the outset of this discussion.

Virtue ethics can seem to veer in the direction of self-centred egoism but in reality, although this ancient model of ethical discourse introduces a significant element of self-cultivation into its musings, this is not to drive consideration away from others but to break down the division between altruism and egoism.[16] Attempting to cultivate a clarity of ethical vision and sound moral motivations through permaculture is not separate from the activities of reduced consumption, caring for living things, sharing knowledge etc. they are inextricably linked.

Much of the 'highly contestable' nature of the more consequentialist approach to the merits of permaculture comes in the form of the impotence and even indulgent nature of 'lifestyle ethics'. As Greg Sharzer suggests in *No Local: Why Small Scale Alternatives Won't Change the World*, this kind of self-provision gardening may well represent just an effort to whitewash alienation, to offer a balm for bourgeois guilt (Sharzer 2012, pp. 100–105). We lucky few can flee to our patches of green, put all the nastiness of global capitalism behind us, and pretend that this seclusion severs us from the cycles of suffering and injustice in which the rest of the world is embroiled. Not only is this lifestyle very passive in its ethical contributions, it is also weak to the point of negligibility: the cogs keep turning anyway.

There are five important responses to this kind of objection to 'localism': (1) Small contributions, even futile contributions can be morally laudable even when offered with knowledge of their impotence. (2) Refusing to engage in an immoral activity, though passive, can be entirely appropriate when more active measures are beyond reach. (3) The primary focus of this recommendation of permaculture is on its usefulness as a mode of moral education and whilst this would be absurd if the activities involved were demonstrably impotent or even wicked in their consequences, that sort of refutation would require just such a demonstration. (4) Permaculture is (as has been said) avowedly holistic and, far from precluding the inclusion of other less locally-focused activities, may well require them. (5) It may also be appropriate to place a particular emphasis on one's more immediate ethical environment: to focus on one's own lot.

With a particular focus on elucidating what is meant here by the appropriateness of emphasizing 'one's more immediate ethical environment' (5), it may be possible to offer a robust response to the localism objection and to simultaneously shed some light upon these other responses (1–4). By focusing on an idea of 'territory' (or 'belonging'), not only can sense be made of why this 'lifestyle ethics' can avoid objections of egoism and bourgeois escapism, but also the way in which justice plays a core role in this symbiotic ethics can be clarified.

Territory ('belonging')

The kind of ethical prioritisation we permit, the kind of discrimination which is intuitively plausible, is not restricted to species (or what has here been discussed in terms of capacities for flourishing or δαίμων), we discriminate also on the basis of 'belonging'. It is not only intuitively right to be more concerned about harming a fox than harming an ant, it is also intuitively right to be more concerned about harming *my* fox, than a stranger.

This discrimination on the basis of 'belonging' can easily be conflated with discrimination on the basis of whether a thing is more or less similar to oneself and with a symbiotic ethics (which incorporates a kind of speciesism based on δαίμων) it will be important to clarify the differences.

'Belonging' means, here, something very similar to the motivation towards 'fellowship', 'communion' or 'solidarity' aforementioned as a sound basis for pursuing rather than avoiding 'negative' emotional states. It is a kind of specialised ἀγάπη in the face of φρόνησις and our own psychological and biological limitations.

When Bernard Williams explains that questioning the permissibility of prioritising the saving of one's own wife is to introduce 'one thought too many' (Williams 1981, p. 18), he is drawing our attention to ethical motivations which are intuitive and at risk of being obliterated by standardising ethical systems like Utilitarianism (*Ibid.*, p. 150). Frankfurt's revision of this parable into terms of 'love' (as opposed to Williams' marriage) may seem pedantic but it permits a focus upon the nature of a particular kind of motivation or virtue and so is useful here (Frankfurt 2004, pp. 36–38). This discussion of 'love' also permits Frankfurt to distinguish this motivation from something which might be a reaction to inherent value:

> As I am construing it, love is not necessarily a response grounded in awareness of the inherent value of its object. It may sometimes arise

like that, but it need not do so. Love may be brought about – in ways that are poorly understood – by a disparate variety of natural causes. It is entirely possible for a person to be caused to love something without noticing its value, or without being at all impressed by its value, or despite recognising that there really is nothing especially valuable about it.

(Ibid., p. 38)

Now if ἀγάπη, compassion/charity/universal love, is understood as a desire for a thing (whether oneself or another) to 'do well', then it is entirely possible to see how this grander virtue, despite its distinct character, can be at the source, in combination with other virtues, of various dispositions. Certainly, this 'love' is at the heart of Schweitzer's indiscriminate desire for all living things to 'do well', for their will to live to remain unhindered as far as possible. Similarly, this motivation (when combined with φρόνησις and direct experience) is vital to a discriminating awareness of different capacities to 'do well' (δαίμων). It is also possible to see that when combined with a kind of honesty, this desire for 'doing well' can be at the core of the appropriateness of sharing in those occasions when any living thing is not flourishing: when it is suffering.

Frankfurt's sense of 'love' is far less broad than these previous uses though, it is, in fact, far more familiar. All of these other kinds of love, even when they discriminate on the basis of capacities or inherent value, are somewhat less personal, they still drive in the direction of perfection and asceticism. Just as Frankfurt says, it is entirely possible to imagine that out of a desire for all things to flourish I am brought to a different kind of *personal* love, but this needn't be so; in fact, the reverse is perhaps more probable and, crucially, more relevant to this current discussion. I am more likely to care about all dogs because I love *my* dog than I am to care about one particular dog because I care about living things in general. I am more likely to be brought to a fuller understanding of the various 'lovablenesses' (δαίμων) of all life by coming to care about particular living things.

It is tempting to imagine that this very familiar kind of affection, of a preference for those to whom we are 'close' is an inclination which can account for the kind of psycho-biological speciesism which has been cobbled together in δαίμων. Indeed, it is this kind of assumption which can lie at the heart of many objections to speciesism: 'you only think a monkey is more important than a trout because the monkey is more like you and this is an arbitrary basis for moral judgements'. This reflects the earlier discussion about 'personhood' and humanoids, with similar analogies to racism being applicable. Of course, this kind of reasoning may well be the origin of some discrimination between different species but the reason for so relentlessly pursuing a novel kind of speciesism is that this superficial basis for discrimination is not ethically sound.

The motivation I have for donating money to a pig sanctuary rather than a salmon sanctuary should be of a different kind to the motivation for buying nice food for *my* pigs. If a single ethical principle were the basis of both my preference for my own pigs and my preference for pigs as opposed to salmon then there would be a sense in which these judgements took place on a single, linear scale and this just seems absurd. My inclination to feed my pigs, to protect them from harm, to be witness and party to their flourishing, does sit on the same scale as my inclination to, say, feed my daughter, but it is somewhat different from my inclination to give refugees food and protect them from harm. The passionate, immediate nature of one inclination and the contemplative, discriminating nature of the other might have led some to believe in the ethical superiority of the latter kind of 'love', and that this removed compassion must oust our irrational favouritisms, but such censorship is far from self-evidently virtuous.[17]

Mary Midgley's inclination to draw a parallel between speciesism and 'familyism' is an understandable one since, not only do both kinds of discrimination seem intuitively correct, they also seem to hold such deep-seated places in our ethical inclinations as to be vital to human wellbeing, as she says:

> Questions about the morality of species preference must certainly be put in the context of the other preferences which people give to those closest to them. These preferences do indeed cause problems. By limiting human charity, they can produce terrible misery. On the other hand they are an absolutely central element in human happiness, and it seems unlikely that we could live at all without them. They are the root from which charity grows.
>
> (Midgely 1983, p. 103)

Yet, there is nothing precluding the drawing of our ethical waters from multiple wells. Williams' aim of protecting our varied and fundamental ethical motivations from the rampaging sterilisation of neatly cohesive and logically consistent moral 'systems' is entirely compatible with Midgley's recognition of the inextricable role these motivations play in 'human happiness'. If these inclinations can be found to coexist (intellectually, emotionally and practically) then an understanding of different kinds of 'love' may help to address some of the difficulties which a single concept encounters. A motivation corresponding to a rich conception of something like 'livingness' (based on a broad idea of capacities for flourishing, psychological and otherwise: 'δαίμων') can account for a hierarchy which places an oak tree above a mouse or an octopus above marmoset (or perhaps a microscopic ecosystem above an individual mammal). A motivation-based solely on 'closeness' will struggle to account for this kind of discrimination. This more familiar ethic based on 'closeness' does, however, seem a far better fit for the appropriateness of having more concern for *my* marmoset rather than some anonymous octopus or *my* mouse rather than an oak tree on the other side of the world. There is some way, perhaps, to do justice to both Midgley *and* Singer.

Here I would recall the earlier discussion of an experience of continuity between my tomatoes and my daughter.[18] Personal affection for both brings to the fore their more basic continuity in δαίμων. I do not, of course, perceive greater importance in my daughter's flourishing than my tomatoes' flourishing simply because my daughter has greater δαίμων, this is also because I love my daughter far more deeply and closely than I do my tomatoes, she belongs to me in a way that the tomatoes cannot. But this second kind of love, this personal affection, attachment and belonging, though it is distinct, comes to illuminate a broader kind of love or regard for livingness in general. So, whether Midgley is correct that this love is the sole 'root from which charity grows' or whether Frankfurt is right that this causal link is not necessary, it may be quite plausible to suggest that personal affection is a *good* source of greater wisdom, if not *the best* source.

Regardless of the accuracy of Midgely's claim on the exclusivity of origin, it may still be observed that her assertion that these affections are 'an absolutely central element in human happiness' seems quite accurate. As has been repeatedly suggested, whether an ascetic ethic can be recommended at all to *anyone* does not alter the probable futility in recommending such an ethic to *everyone*. Indeed, it may well be asserted that to imagine a human (or any living thing for that matter) without belongings, is to imagine a thing no longer living. Now, to jump from personal love to 'belongings' may seem an unfair conceptual leap or conflation but the continuity between what might more commonly be recognised as ownership and the 'love' of Frankfurt is vital to the conception of 'belonging' currently being sought.

At the outset of this chapter, an attempt was made to outline the nature of my experience of my own interests clashing with those of the rats who share my garden. This was and is an experience of overlapping territories, of interests and identities which stretch into both an environment and other living things. They were *my* chickens, that's why I tried to scare the rats away, that is why we fought and why they died.

When a horsefly lands on my arm and drills their mouthpiece into my flesh there is a clear sense of violation and a corresponding clarity in the justification of my unthinkingly violent response. I kill the horsefly. This clarity of justification seems like it may be defined by my own bodily boundaries but the reality of lived identity is very far from such dermatological definition.

There are times when I look at my wife or my daughter and I lose any particular sense of being something other than them. In an embrace their smell and breath are not something which I am not, there is no sharp boundary, indeed there may be times when I am more them than I am me, when I feel their pain (though not in precisely the same way) far more forcefully, far more urgently than I feel my own, when their smiles and my joy are immediate. This needn't be romantic nonsense, nor does it need to be more poetry than sober observation. These occasions do not permanently erase my individuality, nor do they really call that individuality into serious question because without that basis of *me* this experience of continuity would be meaningless, instead these moments of conjunction illuminate the complex and extended nature of my identity or sense of self. Even when this sense of self is extended into a more reflexive, temporal, narrative sense, there is room for fracture and strange losses of continuity. Even a central character is composed of many plot lines.

Perhaps, indeed, the most familiar way in which we encounter this kind of extended identity is temporal. We are concerned about our past and future selves in ways that differ from our concern for our present self but this concern is a nebulous and extended thing. We very naturally think of ourselves as things which are not purely situated in the infinitesimal present moment but instead are spread out in time, we dwell on past wrongs and anticipate future success. Indeed, the moral relevance of these past and potential events is not only proportional to their own magnitude and inherent significance but also how far away they are. Very often, that which happened yesterday or is likely to happen tomorrow is of greater concern than that which happened a decade ago or is certain to happen in the distant future. These classic components of consequentialist calculations are powerful elements of our lived ethical realities and whether this inclination feeds into vice or virtue is of significant ethical concern.

The concept of belonging currently being proposed as integral to well-being would take this kind of temporally extended identity, together with a spatial, material and causal extension, and identify this regard for ourselves with personal affection, with Williams' 'justification' for saving his wife rather than a stranger.

Of course, this is not a novel approach to love and belonging. An ascetic ethic would eschew all such forms of 'attachment' (temporal, material, intellectual, emotional etc.). When it was 'asserted that to imagine a human (or any living thing for that matter) without belongings, is to imagine a thing no longer living' we needn't look very far for just such an example. The Sokushinbutsu were one group of humans who did just this.

Though many tried, only very few succeeded in achieving the self-mummification which these Buddhist monks valourised.[19] This state of 'deathlessness' was (and is) seen as a vindication of their attempts to reach a purer state of existence. The Four Noble Truths which lie at the heart of all Buddhist schools pivot about one piercingly dreadful conception of suffering, of दुःख (Dukkha). दुःख is real and it should and can be escaped. Ἀταραξία, in this view, comes through a severance with the chaos of the material world. The Sokushinbutsu understood this central ethos of Buddhism in the most strikingly direct way and took it to its logical conclusion. The raging chaos of the world, the unfathomable cascade of cause and effect, the dreadful nausea of responsibility in this teeming cesspit of life, the hopeless confusion of a personal identity spread and fractured throughout time and desire. The extension of self and one's own connection with suffering are the same, contract the self and one will be liberated from suffering. It is possible for the human being to become a stone, a distilled, simple and inert mote of existence. Unmoving, unliving, undying. For the best part of a decade you will starve yourself. For the first thousand days eat only seeds and rid your body of all fat and excess flesh. Now progress to eating only bark and roots to starve yourself further and into complete emaciation. The third stage is, little by little, to drink the sap of the urushi tree and a potion of arsenic; this stage will desiccate you, removing all excess moisture. Finally, after years of preparation, you will enter your tomb and cease all consumption, you will drift from this world in a state of complete and absolute meditation, if you have succeeded then your companions will reveal you one thousand days later in a mummified state, you will have become a monument to an escape from belonging. No time, no agency, no ownership. A complete retraction of self into a kernel of responsibility.

This is an end to life. Perhaps Singer would suggest that the Sokushinbutsu were ultimately selfish and that this 'sacrifice' did nothing but service a delusion based on esoteric metaphysics and not upon real ethical concerns. Instead, we should simply understand our responsibilities on the basis of a reasonable and clear appreciation of the agency. An empirically based, statistically informed understanding of our ability to affect events in the world needn't be overwhelmed by the mysterious magnitude of the metaphysical problems surrounding the causal universe and the place of our selves (or 'no-selves') in it. Such cosmic speculation and mystical anxiety are disingenuous. Like the Stoics, let us just try to understand what we *can* do and then do our best. Forget all the finer details about personal wellbeing, the indulgence of luxuries, the inevitabilities of suffering and Wolf's 'strangely barren' asceticisms, all these musings accomplish is the impeding of efforts in genuinely effective altruism.[20]

Singer's suggestion that proximity is morally irrelevant remains a powerful suggestion:

> Once we are all clear about our obligations to rescue the drowning child in front of us, I ask: would it make any difference if the child were far away, in another country perhaps, but similarly in danger of death, and equally within your means to save, at no great cost – and absolutely no danger – to yourself? Virtually all agree that distance and nationality make no moral difference to the situation. I then point out that we are all in that situation of the person passing the shallow pond...
>
> (Singer 1997)

Yet the insight is hollow when stacked against Bernard Williams' wife drowning and it does little to pay service to the complexity of Midgley's suggestion that personal proximity (whether causally or through affections and other associations) is central to human happiness. Certainly, Singer is correct that the inevitability of this impulse is, by itself, morally irrelevant and that its importance as a source of other ethical impulses does not justify its sovereign indulgence in the face of more pressing responsibilities. And yet, Midgley's suggestion that these inclinations are at the core of our being can help to illustrate the way in which a combination of inevitability and seminality helps to shape an understanding of a disposition which, as Bernard Williams suggests, precedes abstract considerations of power.

There is a sense in which my killing of the horsefly is justified not by considerations of what choice amongst many is the best choice but, rather, the way in which my sense of bodily integrity is something which can and should be defended and that to imagine a being which considers the exercise of its own agency as being *entirely* abstracted from those kinds of reactions is to imagine a being which is as desiccated, inhuman and as dead as those Japanese mummies. The proper way to consider the ethical weight of our personal affections is not like the rarified weighing of charitable donations but *more like* the killing of the horsefly.

As has already been intimated, it would be naïve to imagine that agency can be neatly divided into rational and considered actions (which are morally relevant and sovereign) on the one hand, and non-conscious, or barely-conscious dispositions (which can just about be tolerated as long as they don't get in the way) on the other. More or less abstract considerations do certainly feed into ethical conduct and so do our senses of personal responsibility due to affections and proximity. This is not just some kind of congenital foundation which can be disposed of when 'better reasons' are conceived of, thick psychology means that personal proximity *is* ethically salient.

What is perhaps most striking in permaculture is how this ethical salience (the sense of justification in taking direct responsibility for the lives most closely related to my own) is inseparable from a sense of power and agency exercised directly in that same sphere of responsibility. This may seem to be almost tautological: power or agency being related to personal responsibility and affection, but what is demonstrated through permaculture is the way in which a clear appreciation of one's place in an ethical universe is bound tightly to a sense of one's own practical potency. To be an affective moral deliberator is to ask the question 'what should I do?', and an image of a rational creature suspended in a world of technologies and statistics which enable extremely precise calculations as to the affect one can have on very distant persons and events, may seem to make good sense. It is necessary, however, in order to properly understand the question *'what should I do?'*, to also have a solid appreciation of what is meant by *'what I do'*.

Through an ethics which identifies εὐδαιμονία with σοφία one can perhaps appreciate more fully the vital role a firm sense of personal agency has in leading a good life. The things which are causally and emotionally close to me are, in a very real and tangible sense, the things which, in large part, constitute me *as such*. For me to flourish my family must flourish and my garden must flourish. This is classical alienation writ large (or, indeed, writ small). Each movement of my secateurs is part of a rich and immediate tapestry of 'what I do', of 'doing well', and there is no clear separation between that sense of agency and of an appreciation of 'what I *should* do'. Of course, abstraction and calculation are not banished from this picture, that would just be to replace one fruitless ethical monopoly with another. Indeed, this process of permaculture, of immediate agency and personal responsibility, can help to form a particularly rich conception of justice. An understanding of the means by which others can flourish is enriched and only accurately understood through an appreciation of the way an organism's means of flourishing and its identity suffuse one another. Bodily integrity, freedom of movement, access to food and water, to clean air and open skies, to room for roots and rich soils; all of these things overlap in unending, interdependent and competing systems of flux.

Just as with the earlier discussion of a holistic model of learning, this theory can sound very similar to models of embodied cognition. Indeed, if less emphasis were placed on the cerebral elements of cognition and this kind of philosophy of mind were permitted to be applied to ethics and broader concepts like 'identity', then certain theories of embodied cognition do reflect many of the ideas being suggested here. As Favela and Chemero suggest:

> ...if cognition is truly embodied, then cognition is also extended. We treat 'cognition' as something that systems do and treat the 'animal-environment' as a system. If cognition is something that systems do, and if cognition is embodied in that system, then cognition is something which extends beyond animal boundaries.
>
> (Favela and Chemero 2016, p. 59)

If the previous anti-cerebral (or only semi-psychological) gloss of δαίμων is allowed for here, and 'cognition' is not meant in any strongly rational sense, then this kind of philosophy of mind can easily support an ethic in which personal proximity is given weight. Crucially, this idea of extended identity avoids more complex and contract orientated ethics of duty. It is not that talking about duties and agreements is not compatible with this talk of extended identity, quite the reverse, instead it is a matter of setting this ethical dialogue in a novel form which avoids some of the strictures of previous formulations.

If I base my duties towards, for instance, my pigs, purely on an idea of implicit agreements, or of contracts based on levels of intelligence, power and agency, then I will be treating certain elements of my ethical world with an attention and emphasis which can threaten to undermine or clash with other considerations and, more crucially, conceptually fracture this world in an artificial way. There is a basic sense in which I care for my pigs in a particular way because they are *my pigs*. They are *mine and* they are *pigs*. And when I have a sense that these pigs 'belong' to me this can cover a variety of impressions ranging from ownership to companionship but all of this is founded in a sense of my local sphere of existence. Abstractions from this tangible world of straw beds, buckets of water, tummy rubs and muddy snouts, cabbage white caterpillars, my daughter laughing and early frost curling leaves, will, in isolation, inevitably fail to accurately correspond to or powerfully motivate actions within this cohesive environment.

This use of the concept of belonging or extended identity (or integrity) has much in common with Gaita's suggestion that the idea of 'rights' adds nothing to a discussion of justice, he says:

> Unless an appeal to rights has force to back it, an appreciation of the wrong being protested depends entirely on a spirit of justice in those to whom the appeal is made. That appreciation need not – I think should not – include the concept of rights.
>
> (Gaita 2003, p. 201)

Explaining that I should feed my daughter properly because of some discreet and immaterial contract which was struck at the moment of conception (or birth), does nothing whatsoever to enrich my tangible appreciation that she is *my daughter*. And this understanding of that which is 'of me' is a rich one which comes in degrees; indeed it is, just as with all phenomena discussed here, a matter of interwoven stories which relate to one another in complex directly perceivable ways. I have no clear notion of how this sense of responsibility would alter for those who adopt children, or for those who 'inherit' the children of others. I have no doubt that the dynamic of belonging would be altered (however subtlety or dramatically), but the contributing plotlines, settings, images and characters would all contribute to a new and unique instance of belonging. What is clear, however, is that this sphere of belonging, this territory, is, in some form or another, absolutely necessary, and it has limits.

The ingredients for flourishing are as variable as life itself and, at times, just as bottomless. I am certain that my pigs would do much better if they had more space and if that space included more trees and frequent change. I make sure they have food and clean water. In hot weather, I ensure they have a cool wallow with plenty of water and mud. But they are all different. Some are content with old straw, others enjoy new straw; one is very large and needs lots of food, two are very small and need far less. But I watch them to know how they are, I listen to them when they go to bed, their little chit chat and sudden arguments. Do they have enough space? Are they getting along? Who is in charge? These questions are real and don't need to fall into the barely-conscious obscurity of immediate impressions which has at times dominated the formulation of ethical reflections in this discussion. But these questions are practical and simple, they are achievable and immediately perceivable.

Put the pig in a cage and see the pig disintegrate, put the tree in a cave and see it wither, sow seeds on to concrete and watch them rot. Instead, I put my pigs in woodland watch them play, I allow trees room to spread their roots and branches and I keep my seedbeds well mucked. What permaculture allows me to understand in the most direct of ways, is that I too am one of these lives and that *my* garden itself is the place where I may flourish.

This may seem a trite and very personal conclusion: 'I like permaculture', but that is not altogether what I am saying. Every living thing has its territory and these territories are inevitably interdependent and frequently in competition. What symbiotic ethics reveals is the way in which a living system as a whole requires a balance of countless territories and that these territories frequently subsume one another. Identities contain other identities, stories contain other stories, and the more stories a story contains, the more lives within that life, the greater the δαίμων.

Certain identities foster a greater richness of co-identities. The oak tree is extraordinarily generous in this regard. The pedunculate and sessile oaks support more life forms than any other tree in the British Isles. Thousands of species live in, on and around the oak, it is a world of worlds. The flourishing of the oak tree depends upon and leads to the flourishing of many other species. The crucial fact about permaculture is the practical and immediate way in which one is forced to acknowledge that, if one's garden is to flourish then the human must be like this, the permaculturist must be like an oak tree.

Now, a fully grown oak is, quite usually, an enormous organism. The tree's requirements for light, water and nutrients mean that it and its companions utterly transform the land in which they live. Thick foliage blots out the sun and prevents many other plant species from flourishing beneath; spreading root systems similarly deny other species an opportunity to thrive. And yet because the oak has arrived at this way of life so slowly and because each individual tree takes hundreds of years to reach this state of dominance, far more life thrives within its sphere of influence than is denied an opportunity. So many species have adapted to live within the oak wood because for each niche it takes away four more are added. Light may not reach the floor but a vast and abundant canopy gives a new vista for those plants and animals which can cling to branch and leaf; deep, complex gouges in the oak's bark create a vast surface for lichens, mosses and herds of microorganisms to populate.

When one grows one's own food, when one sows a seed, it becomes apparent that each living thing has a sphere of this sort, an extended identity. Each pea plant needs soil, water and light of just the right kind in order that it might flourish, and so too does each variety and species require its own mixture of factors to call its own; a certain freedom, a certain food. When one approaches this little world of territories from the universal love of Schweitzer, it becomes readily apparent that, although a human must cast its shadow over the land, so too can new places for life open through our actions. It becomes clear that far from the denial of flourishing being required for (or the consequence of) any other organism flourishing, the flourishing of all is, quite generally, a necessary part of the flourishing of the individual.

This is, of course, a quite well-established dictum of not only permaculture but also modern ecology in general. That ecosystems are hugely complex networks of interdependent organisms operating through symbiotic relationships of differing degrees of proximity and that each part is important to the whole.[21] What permaculture offers is the ability to enact this, to perceive it directly through living as one of those organisms in one's own sphere of influence, what the garden offers is an opportunity to fully appreciate the sense in which 'I am life which wills to live, and I exist in the midst of life which wills to live.' And this participation in 'life', in the great δαίμων, establishes a very clear sense of the way in which we are, each of us, things beyond ourselves.

Standardising moral systems can create a picture of a human agent as an isolated, rational ghost, a kind of simple fragment of moral responsibility which is separate from the rest of the world. This kind of ratio-centric moral system can make it difficult to appreciate the importance of and respect due to those with whom we share a world. Do they deliberate? Do they have rights? Are they agents? If we are, instead, able to appreciate the way in which any organism is constituted by its ecological context, that it is a nexus rather than an atom, then the nuances and complexities of justice can make far more sense.

And yet, this vague appreciation of extended organisms as the locus of moral responsibility not only risks ethical vacuity through its breadth, it also begins to sound quite conservative and 'old fashioned'. If living well becomes a matter of giving each its due, of the appropriateness of one organism dominating another as long as it fosters further life, then won't we just end up with a kind of Hobbesian monarchy (albeit a benevolent one)?

Well, perhaps drawing political conclusions in this way isn't altogether wrong, and it certainly goes some way to putting some normative meat on these otherwise sparse metaethical bones.

One means of reaching this kind of normative conclusion with greater clarity will be to attempt a reconciliation of otherwise disparate and seemingly incompatible elements. Schweitzer speaks of perfection, and this sits quite comfortably with the moral realism with which this discussion opened, yet it sits poorly with the messy pragmatism and (albeit virtue-based) almost 'power orientated' ethics of δαίμων speciesism. How can an embrace of the darkness of life be reconciled with a quest for Goodness itself?

Notes

1 Of course, viruses occupy a position on the scale of δαίμων so extreme that they might (and often are) considered not to be living things at all (see Zimmer's [2015, p. 105] *Planet of Viruses*). Since, however, δαίμων is a primarily inclusive concept designed to dissolve the ethical power of well-defined boundaries, this extremity enhances this illustration rather than detracting from it.

2 On the scale of parasitism see A. Dobson et al.'s (2008) *Homage to Linnaeus: How many parasites? How many hosts?*

3 Of course, the example needn't be ancient or biblical. The dichotomy between civilisation (or a desirable environment) and a hostile wilderness which must be tamed or eradicated is sufficiently modern as to be extant (though many of these more recent instantiations take ancient president as their inspiration); see A. A. den Otter's (2012, pp. xxi–xxiii) *Civilising the Wilderness*.

4 Mike Martin identifies Schweitzer's muddle of a dichotomy between absolute ethical values and practical necessity as being a significant failure of his ethical theory (Martin 2007, pp. 21–22).

5 Of course, much could be said about the distinction between 'right' and 'good' (see W. D. Ross' [1930, pp. 10–11] *The Right and The Good*). Suffice to say here that by 'right' I mean to say that which is the correct course of action (based on that which is the virtuous thing to be done, that which is based on the right sorts of motivation) and by 'good' I mean to suggest the kind of world and events which are desirable. The correct, morally laudable course of action may nevertheless be regrettable in many ways and not unremittingly good.

6 As M. W. Martin acknowledges, Schweitzer can seem to be recommending a very narrow kind of ethic with his emphasis on perfection yet this orientation needn't preclude (and in Schweitzer's case does not preclude) the contribution of a wide array of virtuous dispositions in ethical deliberation (Martin 2007, pp. 2–3).

7 An emphasis on ἀγάπη as a key virtue certainly reflects a departure from the classical grounding of this discussion into a more Christian history. Of course, Schweitzer's own thinking was of a Christian nature, but more importantly it is entirely consonant with the rest of this discussion to suggest that a movement or development in the history of philosophy contributed a profoundly important insight. Of course, Hellenes were familiar with the role of ἀγάπη in ethical conduct (no moral creature could be without such a basic awareness) but the rise of Alexander, of Rome and finally the collapse of classical European civilisation encouraged a shift (and contraction) of philosophy which enabled new insights to come to the fore. A reformulation of the virtues may be foremost amongst these Christian contributions to philosophy and is something to be enormously grateful for.

8 It might be claimed that ἀγάπη in its truest form is also holistic, that a universal love for all things is the fullest realisation of ἀγάπη. But even if credence were given to this notion, a universal love is more like a potential than a realised virtue. The saint who could profess such a state would nevertheless find their compassion active only when confronted with particular examples, particular individuals. Certainly, one can ponder, in the abstract, the fate of *all* creatures, but this is still, in an important sense, a particular scenario. To be constantly torn apart by all suffering (past, present and future) and to likewise be absorbed by the joy of its antithesis would be to exercise a virtue which was no longer a recognisably mortal condition: something divine, something unattainable, barely imaginable, something normatively meaningless, the love of gods.

9   The distinction here between 'dispositions' and 'feelings' (with the former giving rise to the latter) is an artificial one and, if taken literally, paints an overly simplistic psychological model of moral character. There is no point at which compassion stops and sadness and joy begin. The division is not psychologically accurate but for the sakes of the above discussion, discussing these things in this way is convenient and the conceptual relationships are unimportant.

10 Teaching raises this sort of ethic to the surface. In my own experience, students can and will ask questions to which one does not know the answer. Given a student's relative lack of knowledge, it is frequently possible to hide a lack of knowledge behind argumentative dissimulation: to make a student think you have answered their question when, in fact, you have not. This can occur in degrees and I have both seen this done and have certainly approached doing it myself. The temptation is very great to create an image of oneself as more knowledgeable than one actually is.

11 Again, a distinction is being made here (between theoretical and practical honesty) for the sake of argumentative convenience. The distinction is an artificial one and is not meant to contravene the overarching model of living-with philosophy. Indeed, the conclusion (that both forms of honesty are ethically equivalent) should be viewed as supporting this underlying metaphilosophical model.

12 One might contrast with this the ideas of Gary Francione (2010, p. 11) as expressed in *The Abolition of Animal Exploitation*.

13 As has already been suggested, this distinction between author and reader is yet another confused dichotomy and would also come into the danger of stretching the literary analogy too far. The kind of synthesis between Aristotelian ethics and literary theory which Ricoeur formulated is certainly very helpful and these are ideas which I have closely followed, but I have attempted to steer as clear as possible from the kind of self-focused, existentialism professed by Ricoeur (Ricoeur 1983, pp. 36–37).

14 It is well to note that the coherence of a single, all inclusive concept of alienation is not necessary for the purposes of outlining the parallels between dealienation and 'amidstness'. Objections like those of Richard Schacht: '... there is no such thing as alienation... But there are myriad alienations' can be accommodated by this current enumeration of types of dealienation (indeed, this kind of objection may support this current division of types). There are different kinds of moral disposition (virtues) which drive these different forms of re-familiarisation, confrontation and conscious efforts towards 'amidstness', and those conceptual unities which have been identified as underlying this model of ethical motivation are sufficiently removed from the concept of alienation to avoid any counter-productive conflation (however fashionable or otherwise such a conflation may be). Part of the point of discussing the garden as a locus for this moral education is to indicate a practical cohesion rather than focusing on a conceptual unity (Schacht 1976, p. 149).

15 To correctly understand the development of permaculture as an idea and practise, it is important to recognise the vital role played by Masanobu Fukuoka. Larry Korn (2015) has been instrumental in bringing Fukuoka's work to the English- speaking world (see L. Korn's *One Straw Revolutionary: The Philosophy and Work of Masanobu Fukuoka*, 2015). There are, of course, a wide range of approaches which may or may not be included under the rubric of 'permaculture'. The practical necessities of sustainable approaches to food production and consumption more generally are the matter of both vague, flimsy 'philosophies' and resource-focused sciences. Laurel Phoenix and Lynn Walter's edited collection *Critical Food Issues: Problems and State-of-the-Art Solutions Worldwide* brings together many of these diverse issues and approaches (Phoenix and Walter [ed.] 2009).

16 R. J. Devettere (2002, pp. 26–27) gives a good summation of this false dichotomy (and 'anachronism') in *Introduction to Virtue Ethics: Insights of the Ancient Greeks*.
17 C. S. Lewis (1960, pp. 115–130), in *The Four Loves*, is inclined to laud charity (ἀγάπη) above all other love (in this case στοργή or φιλία). Of course, Lewis is concerned with the way in which all love relates to god but ultimately he finds ἀγάπη to be the only 'self-sufficient' love.
18 It should be noted that Tim Ingold also recognises this continuity between caring for plants and other animals and raising children. Ingold offers ethnographic accounts which attest to this experience of continuity and he identifies this continuity as being based in an idea of growth more generally. It is certainly tempting to suggest that this idea of growth closely matches the idea of directly perceiving and responding to capacities for flourishing espoused here but justifying the closeness of that match would require another discussion (and perhaps dialogue) (Ingold 2000, pp. 86–87).
19 As described by T. F. Lobetti (2014, pp. 130–136) in *Ascetic Practises in Japanese Religion*.
20 It is important, once again, to take note of the important role Toby Ord and Peter Singer have played in forming this new take on pragmatic, statistically based utilitarianism. Singer (2015, p. 97) notes Ord's role in many places, but particularly in *The Most Good You Can Do: How Effective Altruism Is Changing Ideas About Living Ethically*.
21 More recent developments in ecology include the use of the idea of 'systems thinking' as integral to the definition of life itself, and this represents a development of just this kind of symbiotic understanding. Firtjof Capra and Pier Luigi Luisi (2014, p. 318) expound just this 'biological' theory in *The Systems View of Life: A Unifying Vision*.

8 An effort to outline an attitude of steady attention, poignancy and good humour in the face of death, as constitutive of wisdom

A violet in the youth of primy nature, Forward, not permanent, sweet, not lasting; The perfume and suppliance of a minute; No more.

(Shakespeare, *Hamlet*, 1.3)

Sunt lacrimae rerum et mentem mortalia tangunt.
There are tears for things and mortal things touch the mind.

(Virgil, *Aeneid*, 1:461 ff)

Get ready,
Get Ready to die,
The cherries say.

(Kobayashi Issa)

There is an elephant in the room: gardening is nice. Gardening is nice because one is outside, doing physical exercise and witnessing closely the beauty of the natural world. This brings peace, this brings satisfaction, this brings happiness in a quite non-technical sense.

Of course, 'gardening' is a misleading term for what has been mostly discussed hitherto as 'permaculture'. Pottering about in herbaceous borders has already been discounted as the subject of this discussion for the reason that it does not closely adhere to the living-with premise of this way-of-life philosophy (it would be too much observation and too little participation). Ornamental gardening of the sort which Cooper discusses (and takes as his primary sense of 'garden') is something which only lies at the fringes of this discussion (Cooper 2006, pp. 15–16). When you take a flower or group thereof, with the primary goal of enjoying this thing aesthetically (and it is usually a case of visual enjoyment) it seems plausible that this activity has more in common with other visual arts than it does with the daily grind of subsistence farmers or the manifold ways of life by which humans have and do sustain themselves across our world through interaction with other species.[1]

And yet even these 'gardeners', even those with grand houses and acres of topiary, even those with blousy blooms dripping with herbicides and neat rows of useless shapes and colours, are, in a certain sense 'living with other living things'. So, there is no need to banish such activities from any and all conscionable considerations. The core idea of permaculture described here should encourage an idea of an activity which is rather more than simply pleasant. I am sure that those who have sufficient wealth and time do find similar revelations and peace in their own fruitless gardens, and the two kinds of gardening are by no means mutually exclusive, but the cabbage has rather more to say than the azalea. No doubt there is always some room for pimms on the lawn, but that is *fringe* to symbiotic ethics. Let us imagine, instead, wilted potatoes and hedgerows in the rain.

What then is left of that stupid pleasure in the sun and flower bed, and what 'more' is there?

Another gardener, another whose name I never knew, he had two allotments. Partly retired he now had more time to spend on the allotment. He had joined these two allotments together, twice the space and every inch considered. He had a strange fruit fly problem on his raspberry leaves; he thought perhaps I might know the cause, I didn't.

I have a sense of awe and shame when confronted by good, old gardeners. Every week he would spend many hours at his allotment and just like the others, just like all *real* gardeners whom I have met, and heard, and read, his labour and pain was a quiet thing.

It is worth repeating an early claim made in this discussion: permaculture is not a 'hobby'. This man worked in the hospital, he had wages, and hours, and lunch breaks and holidays. The allotment happens outside of these things but it is no less a place of labour, or at least, it is no less a place of *work* which should be taken seriously.

But an income orientated culture of worth leaves little room for a clear public dialogue about these 'works', so it is done in a stoic spirit and with a largely unspoken camaraderie in this movement 'back to the land'. Here, in this sterile promontory of wealth, this western world of ancient machines, humanity has been torn from a way of life bred in deep millennia and it can only creep back there in the little spaces, in the quiet moments which this mechanisation affords.[2]

It is perhaps unsurprising that Britain should have such a peculiarly fetishised culture of the kitchen garden and that it should (as with so many things valorised in these islands) hark back to the Victorian dream where that wage machine was born.

They call it a 'stiff upper lip', and this spirit of Stoicism and the English country garden certainly brings this current meditation upon life in an English garden far closer to more traditional discussions of classical philosophy as a way of life.[3] The Victorian manifestation of this ethic is most eloquently expressed in Kipling's (1910) *If*:

> If you can keep your head when all about you
> Are losing theirs and blaming it on you,

If you can trust yourself when all men doubt you,
But make allowance for their doubting too;
If you can wait and not be tired by waiting,
Or being lied about, don't deal in lies,
Or being hated, don't give way to hating,
And yet don't look too good, nor talk too wise:
If you can dream – and not make dreams your master;
If you can think – and not make thoughts your aim;
If you can meet with Triumph and Disaster
And treat those two impostors just the same;
If you can bear to hear the truth you've spoken
Twisted by knaves to make a trap for fools,
Or watch the things you gave your life to, broken,
And stoop and build 'em up with worn-out tools:
If you can make one heap of all your winnings
And risk it on one turn of pitch-and-toss,
And lose, and start again at your beginnings
And never breathe a word about your loss;
If you can force your heart and nerve and sinew
To serve your turn long after they are gone,
And so hold on when there is nothing in you
Except the Will which says to them: "Hold on!"
If you can talk with crowds and keep your virtue,
Or walk with Kings – nor lose the common touch,
If neither foes nor loving friends can hurt you,
If all men count with you, but none too much;
If you can fill the unforgiving minute
With sixty seconds' worth of distance run,
Yours is the Earth and everything that's in it,
And – which is more – you'll be a Man, my son.

Perhaps the jingoism and patriarchy of Kipling are unwelcome, but there is something here of the wisdom of which the ancients speak and which I have heard in the voices and stories of permaculturists time and again. Even those with unruly hair and more musky odours, if they truly dig, if they have muck beneath their nails, then there will be something of this quiet strength in them.

And I think it is about death.

Montaigne says 'that to philosophise is to learn how to die'; I think that's true (Montaigne 1580, pp. 61–80).[4]

It is an idea of death which will be at the heart of this final attempt to reconcile the idea of universal but discriminating compassion for all with the recognition of the inevitability of conflict, negative feeling and classical virtue. This synthesis will also tie together the ideas of absolute goodness, balance and compromise expressed at the outset of this discussion through the medium of aesthetic and narrative anthropological philosophy.

It is a steady pace, poignancy and good humour in the face of death which will characterise this ultimate description of wisdom. The hope is that this conception will not only offer a novel and useful way of understanding wisdom and how to achieve it but also something which fits nicely with the classical and intuitive senses of virtue already discussed.

The forgiving minute

'Why did you stop growing your own veg?' I asked a farrier friend, 'I just don't really have the time, it takes a lot of time' came the answer.

And so it goes, pretty generally, with this line of questioning. I explained that this was one of the two answers I get when I ask people who don't grow veg why they do not do so. The other answer (generally from younger interviewees) is that they don't enjoy it or that they aren't good at it (or some combination thereof). I told our farrier friend how and why this answer of preference was not a good answer, how I always feel like saying I don't care if they like it or not and they won't improve if they don't practice (there are always people willing to teach... always).

This suggestion, that growing vegetables was not about whether you liked it or not, or felt competent, that there were moral demands on doing this thing, seemed agreeable to this man who works with horses.

He planned on taking it back up when he retired (or partly retired).

We got to talking about the link between gardening and the elderly. Perhaps it was just that they now had the time, time in retirement in which to indulge this pleasant luxury. But maybe it was something else, perhaps there was some residue of the victory gardens, some sense of the veg garden contributing to good citizenship. A duty, not a pastime. These didn't seem mutually exclusive reasons.

And I could hardly claim that this man who spends his time bent double, in all weathers, at the feet of horses would benefit from the exercise or outdoor time which permaculture gardening provides. Certainly many of the more subtle benefits in cultivating classical virtues and more clearly appreciating the nature of life itself would still be of benefit to a farrier (not to mention the more usual environmental and economic benefits) but the finer details of this philosophy can represent dubious selling points in a tight spot. And aren't we all in a tight spot? Twixt cradle and grave?

This association we had, between old age and gardening, which is integral to the British fetishisation of gardening, may be useful. This association echoes the more universal connection between old age and wisdom and this conjunction between old age, gardening, wisdom and death is far more than mere coincidence.

As with permaculture, and as has already been stated, philosophy can seem like the luxury of those with time on their hands. Truth for its own sake; who can afford such a thing when the basic necessities of life consume all but the merest scraps of our time and energy?

We do find time for certain things though, don't we? Things which we refuse to mechanise and for reasons of virtue keep close, personal and simple? We might call them natural. Perhaps this, as with Kipling's verse, is redolent of an antiquated conservatism. It comes forth in Chesterton's discussion of democracy:

> It is not something analogous to playing the church organ, painting on vellum, discovering the North Pole (that insidious habit), looping the loop, being Astronomer Royal, and so on. For these things we do not wish a man to do at all unless he does them well. It is, on the contrary, a thing analogous to writing one's own love-letters or blowing one's own nose. These things we want a man to do for himself, even if he does them badly. I am not here arguing the truth of any of these conceptions; I know that some moderns are asking to have their wives chosen by scientists, and they may soon be asking, for all I know, to have their noses blown by nurses. I merely say that mankind does recognize these universal human functions...
>
> (Chesterton 1908, p. 44)

And perhaps this vision of old age speaks as much of something social as it does of something biological. These people come from a world in which growing some food is just one of those things which one must do for oneself. There is an expectation that we find time for certain things and that by seeking to delegate these things for the sake of efficiency we lose something important, something which speaks to the classical virtues of respect, of justice, of courage.

Indeed, this harking back to an age of no-nonsense, hard-working, self-respecting partly self-sufficient people is at the heart of the permaculture movement. An author on a par with Fukuoka in this movement (perhaps even more influential) is John Seymour. It was Seymour's *The New Complete Book of Self-Sufficiency* which acted as a catalyst for thousands of people to join this 'back to the land' movement during the 70s (Seymour 1976). It was, indeed, the book which most influenced my own initiation into permaculture. Seymour's account of self-sufficiency, apart from being eminently practical, is peppered with reminiscences of a time in which some level of self-sufficiency was entirely ubiquitous and upon parts of the world where, for young and old, this remains the norm:

> The country garden of my childhood was a mixture of vegetables, flowers, soft fruit, tree fruit (oh, those greengages!) and very often tame rabbits, almost certainly a hen run, often pigeons, and often ferrets. It was

a very beautiful place indeed. Now, alas, it has disappeared under a useless velvety lawn and a lot of silly bedding plants and hardy perennials.

(*Ibid.,* p. 40)

Seymour's suggestions and life have been the target of some criticism, and
perhaps justifiably so. Monty Don (another paragon of the gardening life),
has voiced his own discontents with Seymour and the ideas he spawned (Don
2016, p. 17). Don is concerned that the more zealous and naive of Seymour's
followers have an all or nothing attitude and that 'self-sufficiency' should
be replaced with a more moderate concept of 'self-provision'. And this difference, between complete, revolutionary self-sufficiency and growing some
vegetables in your garden also seems to echo the characteristics of hurried,
foolhardy youth and *patient*, wise old age.

It should be emphasised that what is not being claimed here is that the
elderly are all-wise and the young all foolish, nor is any kind of empirical
claim being made about trends in wisdom and foolishness and their correlation with age, rather, what is of interest are *established associations* ('stories'
as it were) and whether these associations can cast some light on the concept of wisdom being described here and its association with gardening.[5]
Even were these ideals of youth and old age entirely fictitious, mere myths
(and this entire absence of correlation seems just as implausible as a precise
match) they would still be of some use in describing the nature of wisdom.
For, there seems to be yet another internal contradiction afoot, one which
these associations may illuminate.

The kind of austere, moralistic demands of the good-old-days appear to
make a poor match for the pragmatic, laissez-faire compromises of planting the odd bean if you have a spare half-hour at the weekend. It is easy
to see how an idea of gardening and 'The Good Life' hives off into camps
of bitter, garden centre scouring, Tories on the one side and twinkly-eyed,
yoghurt-weavers on the other (the term 'permaculture is associated far more
with the latter). Quite a gulf lies between these foes. Time is the resource
they distribute differently; one group gives it all, the other offers only the
final scraps.

It would be absurd (and quite immoral) for an academic to brandish
moral expertise in the face of those who work extreme hours for little finan-
cial reward compared to those in education. To recommend a philosophy
with no mind to practical reality is (as has already been claimed as a central
premise of this treatise) not only immoral but also futile. Certainly, one can
imagine a world (as an idea or thought experiment) in which everyone has
time for lots of gardening and recommend just such a system to future gen-
erations. Apart from being of little immediate practical value, however, this
kind of musing would also fail to do justice to the sense in which *our time is
always limited.* Of course, it may be possible to simply take account of differing amounts of 'free time' (which probably means something like: time not
spent making money) and suggest that those with very little should spend

less time gardening whilst those with more should spend more. What may be more powerful, though, is the elucidation of a way of thinking about time which compliments the virtue-driven demand to grow our own food rather than rationing that demand. It is a way of thinking about time (in the not exclusively or highly cerebral sense of 'thinking about' which this discussion has frequently employed) which these archetypes of old age, gardening and wisdom can help illustrate. It is a correct attitude towards time which can assist both Tory and Hippie, overworked nurse and 'wilfully' unemployed. The garden is not just a place to spend time, but a place to learn about how time *should* be 'spent'.

The curious thing about our idealised old person is that they simultaneously have more time and less time and it doesn't seem to be their retirement which is conceptually crucial to the way in which they dig for victory.

As I watched my own grandparents in the garden it became apparent how much harder this task was for them than it is for me. They stooped to weed a patch of ground and their bones creaked under the strain (though I cannot claim to be completely creak-free). They planted a seed without any confidence that they would live long enough to eat the fruits (indeed, in one case, they did not). Each task would take many times longer for them than it would for me and yet I, I from whom death seems so distant, would worry about how to fit this task in here, and that task in there. My future spreads out before me and each decade, year, month and moment become squeezed so tight by a sense of anticipation and expectation that by the time it is upon me it has slipped from my grasp without notice. Tomorrow hurtles towards me with such ferocious speed that I turn my gaze elsewhere so as to avoid its searing inevitability. And yet with those for whom the reality of death is (at least temporally) far nearer, there can be a reversal of this urgency.

There is a sense in which these people grow vegetables not only because they have time and that it is pleasant but because that is just what good people do. The virtues already enumerated which can be cultivated and enacted through self-provision can and are demonstrated by cultures and populations both past and present. These kinds of examples, of allotmenteers and aged victory diggers could and should make for a compelling means of demonstrating the value of this way of life. Yet there is more to this conjunction of age, wisdom and gardening; there is a means of understanding how we should conceive of time and how we 'use' it.

I saw a young man give a reading in a church. Afterwards, he explained to the priest that he had never done this before and that he was hugely anxious about his performance. The priest, a much older man, gently advised that slowing down would be a good idea next time. The young man had anticipated this problem and had even interspersed his script with reminders to slow down. 'It comes with time' explained the priest.

Students do this too; when giving presentations they will fail to manage their pace, they will lose track of time. Perhaps all of us do this sort of thing. Why is it difficult to slow down? Why is it so hard to take a breath and survey that which lies before us? And what if death were closer? What if I were told that I had a decade left? A year? A month? A Week? Would I similarly press these last few increments of time into an optimum reward? Is this what Kipling's 'man' must do? To 'fill the unforgiving minute with sixty seconds worth of distance run'? Perhaps this is what he means, to squeeze our time dry. If so, it sits poorly with the other sentiments he expresses.

A year after Kipling's poem was published, W. H. Davies (1911) offered his own take on this subject in *Leisure*:

> What is this life if, full of care,
> We have no time to stand and stare.
> No time to stand beneath the boughs
> And stare as long as sheep or cows.
> No time to see, when woods we pass,
> Where squirrels hide their nuts in grass.
> No time to see, in broad daylight,
> Streams full of stars, like skies at night.
> No time to turn at Beauty's glance,
> And watch her feet, how they can dance.
> No time to wait till her mouth can
> Enrich that smile her eyes began.
> A poor life this if, full of care,
> We have no time to stand and stare.

There is some common wisdom here, between Kipling and Davies. I have seen it in permaculture.

Kipling's man is solid and quiet, Davies' life is still and patient.

In the chaos of a winter storm a naked oak tree will sway and creak, it will snap and fray. The frosts will enter its wounds and prize them open. The spring brings new life and with this come a thousand tiny mouths, each mouth more hungry than the last. In the heat of summer, the disease will fester on the tips of leaves which have escaped the ravages of these unseen mouths and autumn urges this titan onward again, down into death, forward into life. And after the winter storms return, in the stillness of a cold morning, the 'unforgiving minute' will be counted out by single drips from a gnarled and mossy limb.

That's the thing with time: it is a many-faced monster.

I will watch a bee at work, a thousand bees at work, and I will wonder at their frantic industry. Flower after the flower is examined and utilised, each moment is a moment of action. And yet the activity of these creatures seems right, it is not incongruous with the monolithic, ponderousness of the trees or the earth itself. The bees and a thousand other insects certainly run at a different pace from the soil, the vegetables, the trees, but these paces are complimentary. Indeed there is a dance, just as Davies says, and there is something vital and wise (which is to say capable of informing virtue as opposed to itself necessarily being virtuous) in the way each organism, whether moving in quickstep or a barely perceptible sway, moves together with its fellow dancers.

So why not be the bee? Why not understand our place as that of the fast-moving creature amidst a slow world? And what does this have to do with our sense of mortality and old age anyway?

One answer could be that we certainly can be the bee, sometimes, because sometimes that's what's called for. Any idea of wisdom which necessitated an unceasingly slow pace to all activities would not be wisdom at all but foolishness. Some laudable activities demand speed, they demand urgency. Many of the most obviously selfless acts are those which take place in sudden, unconsidered fits of activity. No thought, barely any sense of intention, just action. Diving into a river to save a drowning child or speaking up in defence of a worthy cause which is under attack, these kinds of the act could almost stand as definitions of courage. Even were the examples less dramatic and confined to more prosaic and practical matters, fast activity is still often appropriate. Self-provision and life lived with other living things afford plenty of occasions for reinforcing this more practical demand for speed. Changes in weather often demand sudden action. One must, indeed, make hay whilst the sun shines. So why, then, with all of these quite intuitively compelling instances of laudable rapid action, should this link between old age, wisdom and slow, still patience persist?

Perhaps it is just a misleading association: a cultural mistake. For one thing, this talk of 'rapid' and 'slow' action may fail to accurately convey the sense in which different kinds of 'quick' activity constitute very different kinds of psychological, conceptual and moral phenomena. Trying to fit many activities into a day and rushing from one activity to another represents a very different sort of activity from split-second decisions made in the heat of the moment, and also from planned but physically rapid activities like sporting activities or exercise. When subjected to greater analytical scrutiny there may be nothing of importance (nothing ethically relevant) to tie these disparate 'fast activities' together. Rather than attempting to delineate these different kinds of activity in an attempt to establish their divisions and permutations, however, it would be far more charitable and fruitful to concentrate on that aspect of 'slowness' which is most relevant and those activities which pertain to this sense.

Davies' life, 'full of care', is not a life which is 'careful'. The life Davies imagines is a life lived without *attention* paid to worthwhile moral concerns, of being distracted by concerns, by worries, which may seem important but which, in fact, when considered carefully and properly, are not so important. This raises again the earlier effort to reconcile Aristotle and Plato's differing approaches to the subject of wisdom through a concept of an appreciation of importance. There is a sense in which 'full of care' contrasts directly with 'careful', proper attention as opposed to improper worry, and it is this 'carefulness' which is synonymous with a steady, slow and gradual activity, something done 'in good time'.

Here we can find conjunction between Kipling's unforgiving minute and Davies' 'no time'. Kipling's sixty seconds stands amidst a list which is full of opposing forces, a list of virtues which sees his man battered side to side by forces of fortune, society and temptation. The middle ground is maintained between these forces in a steady pace to match his meter. Like a metronome or a counted breath, each move comes in the face of opposing forces, a course, like that of Odysseus, steered along a finely balanced path. And all of this is achieved through its own internal force, a kind of restraint and perspective: a stepping back. Whether a force is a push or a pull the internal force counsels a kind of caution, a distributed carefulness.

This is the same practice which was identified with anthropological philosophy, this being directly involved and at the same time withdrawn. Indeed, this is the peculiar paradox which has been a constant theme of this attempt to describe the nature of wisdom by symbiotic ethics; it is that balancing of the seemingly contradictory principles of detail and breadth. Simultaneously paying close attention and allowing for the widest possible picture: a squinting focus through a lens and a wide-eyed scan of the horizon. To focus on the detail of that which is most important and to do so in a way which is not only aware of a wider scheme but a way by which this wider awareness is integral to this focus. As was discussed in relation to Aristotle and Plato's discussion of wisdom (σοφία), a simple focus upon important things would not be true wisdom (always excluding its contrary as itself being an 'important thing'), for it would fail to situate these things in relation to their context and therefore any correct focus would be essentially accidental and fragile (a true belief but not a *justified*, true belief). Simply having a broad view, a cosmic view, would similarly fail to qualify as wisdom since our human condition requires that the most important things (moral insights) are acted upon accordingly (φρόνησις and σοφία).

The virtuous manner of treating and viewing time (which might, perhaps loosely, be identified with the virtue of patience) may owe its association with an idealised vision of old age to just this combination of focus through broad perspective and broad perspective through focus. Careful attention to detail and prioritisation of the small, common but important things in life may seem a natural consequence of the far-reaching experience which this old person would have accrued in their lifetime. Time enough to see mistakes repeated, for regrets to be born out and each act and object to fit more clearly in its place. And yet, there is another boundary, another force at work in this wise-slowness, this care and attention.

Change is inevitable, ubiquitous and vital. Sudden change, slow change, painful change, pleasurable change, beneficial change, harmful change.

Our ideal old age carries not only an experience of life (and the knowledge this affords) but also a chance to greater appreciate the nature of this ubiquity of change and the variety and nature of change as such. As much as time itself can be experienced in the abstract, this wrinkly archetype has an engrained understanding of this constant. By the very nature of this character, they have, through good fortune (and perhaps some design) come to experience the passing away of their own self in a way which is, in a sense, 'seemly'. They are dying slowly, drifting away in such a fashion that mirrors the way the rest of the world moves. Change is death, change is the tempo of the universe and life itself moves at a certain rate, to grow old is to physically engage in this process of living and dying.

The concept which links this ideal old age, the correct way of viewing and treating time, and life in the permaculture garden, is *decay*. These gardeners, you'll find, permaculturists, are experts in and enthusiasts of decay.

Death is rarely a clearly defined event. Just as with δαίμων being a thing which is more or less living, so too does death come in increments. We, as things of much δαίμων, can become used to thinking about death in a very dramatic sort of way. Movement, heat, sound, when these are gone then life has ceased. Even those of us who have other animals prominently in our lives will know the shocking sense of death in the touch of a corpse. It is a strange and alien thing, a world away from the vibrantly living being. And yet, many of us know also that contrary experience of being unsure, of life and death hovering in close companionship, allowing for little certainty (that certainty conventional philosophy craves). Plants give a constant reminder of this death-life. Without the rapidity and vibrancy of animal δαίμων, plants will often appear to be dead only to hold, deep within their withered crust, some green signs of moisture and new life. Vegetative reproduction, the activity of taking cuttings from plants and propagating them into new plants, holds a similar sense of death-life. A severed limb, seemingly a thing destined for immediate corruption, when given the right conditions, will flourish into fresh growth: rebirth.

Yet there is a thing which is neither plant nor animal and both at the same time, a thing which is the ultimate crucible of death-life, the baseline of δαίμων: *compost* is the pride and joy of the permaculturist.

To the uninitiated compost may seem to be a totally inanimate thing, beyond merely dead it is the point at which living things have become so far from life, so far from thriving individuality through this corrupted mixture of detritus, that they now constitute a kind of elemental or mineral substance. Like fire, air or water this stuff is a mere matter, it is earth. And yet how wrong this view would be. The mind of the philosopher, always in the second glance, the mind of the gardener-poet, seeker of wisdom, finds here a steaming jungle of microscopic life. Even to the naked eye compost is a busy thing. The visible signs of bacteria and their appreciable heat are static enough, but a huge range of invertebrates play an enormous role in the decomposition of organic matter. Chief amongst these beings, at least in the eyes of permaculture, are the worms.

Of course, 'worms' is far too generic a term to be of any real biological significance when it comes to the processes of decomposition since there are so many species which, both locally and globally, occupy a range of niches in the processing and redistribution of dead, dying and living matter.[6] And yet, whether it is a meaty earthworm in the cold soil or a sleek tiger worm sliding through steaming muck, these beings are often the visible sign of wellbeing which permaculturists seek and which, despite their variety, offer a sign of continuity in health between the freshest dung and the oldest of soils. When soil or muck is prized open (as infrequently as possible), what one looks for is worms; more worms mean greater soil health, greater soil health means more vegetables. And despite the vibrancy and skittish, otherworldly haste of the mites, ants, centipedes, nematodes, fruit flies and other invertebrates which populate rotting, organic matter, the worms inevitably bind these lesser dances into a great, steady, throbbing rhythm of life. The worms and their dark kingdom beat out the drum to which all life must move. The primordial ooze upon which the worms subsist, the bacterial and fungal slime whence all have come and whither all must return, is the alpha and omega of life itself; the worms show us its health.

What this close familiarity with compost and worms can offer is a real sense of the pace at which life, because of the natural rate at which things decompose, must move. If things die faster than they decay, or live faster than they decay, then that is when problems arise. If vegetables are harvested at a rate greater than that at which nutrients are returned to the soil through these miniature ecosystems of decomposition then life becomes thin and threadbare, the supply lines are overstretched and the chain comes undone. Similarly, the system breaks down when too much matter, too much death, is introduced. Many gardeners are familiar with this latter problem, and the horror of acrid piles of (bad) slime in a compost heap overwhelmed and unable to breathe.

In the most prosaic sense, all of this talk about compost and worms highlights a notable feature about permaculturists which is often lacking from those who do not grow: the growers smile at muck. And this general good humour about muckiness and 'creepy crawlies' is not *only* (for it is this also) a simple, meek, kind-hearted acceptance of things in which other people find cause for revulsion. This embrace of muck is founded on a deep sense of the vital role which these small, steady, humble things play in the grand scheme and the necessarily close relationship between death and life.

This understanding need not be particularly intellectual. Simply by regularly handling this matter which is an intimate and inextricable mixture of death and life, and gaining a keen sense of its importance to the health of all things, and of the slow and steady way in which it develops and decays over seasons and years, one can gain a very direct sense of one's own place in this dance of death-life. The reality of one's status as 'food for worms' may fill some with pure dread, but to this dread permaculture adds joy: 'Oh! To be food for worms!'

Again, as with the stoic resilience of Kipling's 'If', this familiarity with, acceptance, and even celebration of those things which might more commonly be regarded as lowly and repulsive, sits well with Hellenistic traditions of philosophy as a way of life. It is worth repeating that most insightful of Marcus Aurelius' meditations:

> And so, if a man has sensibility and a deeper insight into the workings of the universe, scarcely anything, though it exist only as a secondary consequence to something else, but will seem to him to form in its own way a pleasing adjunct to the whole. And he will look on the actual gaping jaws of wild beasts with no less pleasure than the representations of them by limners and modellers; and he will be able to see in the aged of either sex a mature, prime and comely ripeness and, gaze with chaste eyes upon the alluring loveliness of the young. And many such things there are which do not appeal to everyone, but will come to him alone who is genuinely intimate with nature and her works.
>
> (M. Aurelius Antoninus, *Meditations*, §3:2:3)

It is a species of uncommon attention which the emperor counsels. When one sees the whole one can see how important the small, 'ugly', hitherto insignificant things really are.

And it is not just the Stoics with whom this philosophy chimes. This theme of finding that which is great in that which is lowly is echoed throughout the classical tradition. It may even be tempting to find here the central doctrine of Diogenes and his 'dog-people'. With their insistence on eschewing social norms in favour of lives lived in filth and base, animal-like behaviour, the Cynics exclusively and uncompromisingly sought wisdom in the most insalubrious of ways. And, of course, Socrates' trial is never far from either Marcus Aurelius' wild beasts or Diogenes' dogs. As Ian Cutler recognises in his discussion of the Cynics, despite the extreme ascetic form which the Cynic practice took, the humility of Socrates is common to both these vagabonds and the more sociable Stoics (Cutler 2005, p. 13).

More importantly, than Greek precedent is the fact that this insight is just as common and intuitive as the link between age and wisdom. An awareness of absence, of limitation and full extent, grants the perspective necessary to appreciate the importance of things and, more often than not, things which seemed unimportant whilst within are shown to be highly important when viewed from without. This could be as simple as the truism that people tend not to appreciate what they have until they don't have it, or (more to the flavour of this current topic) the way in which a near view of death (ones own or another's) can cause people to reevaluate their priorities and find, in a strangely surprising way, that small, otherwise mundane things are the truly precious things.

It is indeed (in an echo of Susan Wolf) *strangely surprising*. Strange, not really because of the ubiquity and intuitiveness of this folk-wisdom, but because it is always shocking to find that when grand facades are shattered, when mighty dreams crumble as all things must, it is in the rubble of this wreck, in its dust, that real beauty can be found. It is shocking because silence is shocking when all about is noise and bluster. Socrates' accusers are full of bluster, they are so confident in their own way of life that they progress along their narrow path in a constant state of acceleration. It seems to them that their way is obvious, that the task is transparent however littered by obstacles it may be. It seems as though the best way through an obstacle is to accelerate, even more, to blast through and onward. So why wait? Why question? It can be no surprise that charging through life in this way (full of care) leaves no time to either gain a sense of the grand scale of things, to step back and see the whole picture or indeed to pay attention to the details and small beauties.

Compost has it all. Compost marries life and death in such a way that a grand perspective is inevitable. A sense of creeping and inevitable dissolution suffuses the vitality which compost encompasses and bestows. The quick and the dead pivot about yet another infinitesimal fulcrum, an impossible point upon which the distinction between living and dead depends and in which this distinction is irrelevant. Even the ancient trees depend upon this stratum and to it, they will return. It is composed of them, dark and loamy, dead leaves and rootlets, rotted bark millennia old, and rocks older still: Earth. Not only does compost engender a sense of these grand, cosmic and terminal things it is also, of course, a world of miniature detail. To understand the virtues of compost or soil, one must get down and close, pull it apart with one's hands and inspect the life within, the details of the grain, the identity of the matter, the scent it gives. The broad view and the focused: both withdraw from the swift hubbub, the clean world of money and men, and permit us to see things as they truly are.

Dread and joy

One might fairly describe this slowness as 'patience', or perhaps 'attention' ('temperance' may also fit the bill): a willingness to give time to the unfolding of important things. It might also be observed that, as with the other virtues which go towards a realisation of the master virtue (wisdom: the union of virtues), 'patience' also must wrestle with other virtues. It has already been explicitly acknowledged that certain courageous acts may require an unthinking speed of action, and it has also been acknowledged that different kinds of speed (or haste) may well occupy different moral and psychological statuses. A quick calculation in a moment of difficulty may well result in great advantage. The swift processing of information may mean that mere seconds of deliberation is equivalent to another creature spending an aeon considering an object or event: one woman's five minutes is another woman's hour.

So, this virtue must line up with the others, and through that balancing act which has already been described (something calculated, observed, learned and intuitive) even the virtue of finding the rightful time and place must find its right time and place.

There are two points which must arise from this observation. Firstly, the kind of harmonious dance, the finding of pace and rhythm with the natural world which has been attributed to 'patience' is crucial and must inform any description of this virtue. Secondly, this virtue (despite being one of many parts which combine to form wisdom) permits us to view the characteristics of wisdom which are more than simply the sum of its unified parts.

Behind everything said so far in this discussion of wisdom has been something hitherto unspoken.

'Mono no aware' is a Japanese phrase which is often associated with Virgil's '(Sunt) lacrimae rerum'. '(There are) tears for/of things'.[7] The ambiguity of Virgil's language here is wonderfully expressive of the relationship of learning by doing (participant observation) which has been identified here with good philosophy, and; not necessarily in any particular realm but in the world as such.[8] Is the pathos native to me or to the world, or does the pathos itself demonstrate the fallacy of this dichotomy? Indeed, a certain kind of ambiguity, or indeterminacy, is also crucial to the Japanese use of 'mono no aware': 'aware' (ah-wah-re) can be sadness or joy.[9] What is core to both phrases is a sense of the emotional impact which brokenness, tragedy or just change should have upon us.

It would be fair to equate much of the content of this concept (or group of concepts) to an attempt to deal with the cognitive, aesthetic and ethical dissonance arising from a sense of how things should be and an awareness of how things are: a problem of evil, as it were. The suggestion is, loosely, that when one can hold on to both a sense of what is good in life and the inevitability of dissolution and suffering, one will find that a state of simultaneous sadness and joy is meaningful and appropriate. It is this concept, this attitude of sombre contentment, which was reflected early on in Socrates' smile, the smile of wisdom, and it is this quiet thing which has guided the discussion largely unseen.

So, the suggestion is this: wisdom must be a mixture of different virtues. Different virtues place emphasis on different things which are important. Wisdom is the activity of combining these virtues and weighing their respective values against one another when necessary and finding the best admixture. This practice and judgement are achieved by enacting these different virtues and learning from as broad a range of contexts as possible in which they are called for in oneself and reflected in others (be they human or, as is often more informative, non-human). A perfect amalgam of all virtues fully realised is both practically and conceptually impossible. So, by the pursuit of wisdom it becomes apparent that not only are valuable things limited but so too are the virtues by which those objects are pursued and, although these virtues may be tied together and defined by a unifying principle of 'The Good' (goodness as such), wisdom is not only limited to being an approximation of this goodness, it is also definitively characterised by this approximateness.

There is something a bit contradictory here, an element of the incommensurable, and yet, as was suggested at the outset of this discussion, the accommodation of such contradictions is itself an important part of wisdom. The value of wisdom lies in the degree to which it succeeds in judging appropriately (by observing and learning) and acting accordingly to all those things in life which are most important (those things which make ethical demands upon us). And yet, in order that the greatest degree of success might be achieved one must come to embrace (in a certain sense, for it is a mitigated embrace) the inevitability of failure. To wish this failure away (which would seem very similar to a desire for success) would reflect a hubris entirely at odds with the attention, restraint and humility necessary for wisdom. And so, even at this core of wisdom, another seeming incompatibility must be entertained. Like Socrates' 'human wisdom', the desire for great wisdom requires (indeed, is partly constituted by) contentment with imperfect wisdom.

Cherry blossom does not have an exclusive claim on the teaching of mono no aware. Of course, no suggestion to this effect is inherent in the Japanese love of the cherries, it is more an epitome or convenient conflation. Indeed, the achievement of a sense of transitoriness in all things and the state of being moved to a simultaneous joy and sadness by that sense (mono no aware) is associated with the changing of the seasons quite generally. Nor is this being moved by the flux of the natural world exclusive to Japanese aesthetics.[10] What may be worth noting about the Japanese tradition, however, is the manner in which finding time to appreciate the flowers has become an important cultural staple.[11] Taking a picnic under the trees when they are in bloom is seen as an important thing to do and perhaps there is some collective wisdom in this. What is certain is that the flowers of many species in the Rose family (amongst which the cherries are counted) lend themselves particularly well to the kind of stopping, standing and staring which Davies finds important. The brief, fragile and delicate beauty of these blooms demands that distractions and clumsy movements must be set aside if their virtues stand any chance of being appreciated. Almost as soon as the flower is full, its petals drift into the wind and are gone.

I would nominate the hawthorn as an able alternative to the cherry in teaching a sense of the tears of things.

I know that people regularly fail to notice the mayflower. Cars speed along past hedgerows which, for a short time in spring, are heavy with pinkish-white, like a wall of candy floss snow. And the petals to conform to fleeting type as they are caught in the breeze. But they are smaller than the cherry's petal and these thorn filled zephyrs will be peppered with swarms of confetti so fine that they can seem like flecks of ash delivered from a distant, unknown cataclysm. For me, this raises the thorn above the cherry, this rumour of weddings and conflagrations. The cherries are undoubtedly delicate but their fragility is sometimes too obvious, too tailored to picnic ease. The thorns are dark creatures. They smell like dead things. As a child, I would delight at the confusion on people's faces after I had asked them to smell the mayflower. They are not sure if it is pleasant or not. There is a soft, nauseating, fleshy sweetness to the flower. Somehow the smell achieves a weight and lightness which unsettles something deep in both brains and belly. The fishy edge has also been associated with sex.[12] Triethylamine (TEA), the compound which gives mayflower its discomforting perfume, is also exuded by the recently deceased, and the closely related Trimethylamine (TMA) causes the smell of some rotting fish and vaginal discharge.[13]

Hawthorns cut a particularly ragged figure in their winter nakedness. On the high ground they relent to the cold air so dramatically that their figures, like spider pennants, form cruel exaggerations of the harsh wind, their witch-fingers stretching out in frozen supplication. And behind the soft, pink-stained blankets of spring, the black labyrinth lurks, festooned with crazy teeth. Pre-Christian traditions echo in faerie associations links with the other world, with holy wells and fate-twisting powers.[14] I can entirely sympathise with these dreamy notions, for I know of nothing more elfish, more betweenish, than the Hawthorn.

So, it is not only the fleeting beauty of its blossoms which can help us sense the power of change in all of life but also the perpetual wyrdness of the hawthorn, its uneasy marriage of life and death.

But flowers are important. It can be hard for a bleak skeleton of a thing to catch precious attention; thorns can seem like something to avoid rather than dwell upon. So, let the flowers do the marketing and let their sudden deaths be a reminder. Let this quick succession melt into near simultaneity of life and death to the extent that the elation at one and disappointment at the other can meld together. By stopping to pay attention to the flowers, people have, very importantly, *stopped to pay attention*.

It does not matter how quick someone is, in thought or deed, the flowers open and fall at their own pace. And this is the lesson: like Murdoch, and Weil before her, the otherness towards which attention is paid, upon which attention is set, is utterly key to this virtue. Internal pace must melt away if real attention is to be achieved, it is a kind of surrender to the value beyond oneself. To push or pull, to carry on, would be to fail. Perhaps this too is why the blossoms are so insightful, for they dissolve into the wind so readily, no sooner do they realise their fullest potential than do they offer themselves up to the medium of their destruction. As Weil suggests:

> Pure, intuitive attention is the only source of perfectly beautiful art, truly original and brilliant scientific discovery, of philosophy which truly aspires to wisdom, and of true practical love of one's neighbour.
>
> (Weil 1941, p. 273)

Of all discrete virtues (which is to say those virtues which are necessary but not sufficient conditions of wisdom), this attention comes closest (or perhaps shares a similar status with φρόνησις) to being a practical guide in the realisation of wisdom. And really this is nothing surprising. Wisdom has been characterised as primarily being a process of learning (improvement by coming to understand and acting accordingly) and careful attention is certainly an intuitive part of good learning. Teachers know this well enough, and since we have all been pupils of some shape or form, familiarity with the vital relationship between learning and paying attention is easy to recognise. Yet how many of us neglect this lesson? Philosophy (and symbiotic ethics) is (or should be) just the practice of not neglecting it.

The philosopher is the one who does not turn away, who pays attention. And, in paying attention, finds that there is so very much which matters.

I was talking to the village vicar and explaining how the impact of our cat dying takes on a different character for us since, when you live with lots of animals, you come to be very well-practised in death. Naturally enough the vicar took this as the suggestion that we have become, in a quite usual kind of way, desensitised to death and the loss of those about whom we care. I tried to explain that this is not what I meant. I am not sure I did a terribly good job of conveying the sense of 'well practiced in death' which I truly meant but I attempted to offer a bit of Gatia's insight on the difference between accurate and erroneous sentiment. We are still sentimental, just not *merely* sentimental. Because there is a sentiment which is the most crucial of all sentiments, the *'hinge'* sentiment as it were, that which Schweitzer correctly identifies as the core of all ethics: love, the knowledge that life and its flourishing matters. The vicar pointed out that people in the country tend to be more robust in this sort of way and our conversation turned to how I have found that too many 'country people' become callous and uncaring. Unable to hold on to the enormity of life and death, the sheer scale of how much there is which *does matter*; they throw away their caring and take on a sardonic bitterness towards death, even a perverse pleasure. Not willing to entertain the emotional and intellectual magnitude of both life and death, instead they become a slave to death alone and the creeping inevitability of all destruction becomes the only tune to which they will dance. Pitch hearts I have seen in ruddy faces; icy eyes set like empty wells on cheeks veiny with the poison of ten thousand brandies.

Yet, as has been noted, love (perhaps some combination of universal compassion and proximal affection) may well make itself known as the primus inter pares amongst the virtues, but the various directions in which it pulls us (to all the world and to our home and own) can become an overwhelming and vague collection of impulses, something which threatens self-destruction rather than self-fulfilment. If the forces of love(s) are to be combined in any meaningful and successful way, then a relationship must be developed between oneself and the world which permits an equilibrium between self and world, learner and learned and lover and beloved.

Weil imagines that this balance, this successful acceptance of love, does itself constitute a kind of perfection: 'there exists a focal point of greatness where the genius creating beauty, the genius revealing truth, heroism and holiness are indistinguishable' (Weil 1943, p. 229). It may be imagined that Weil's 'genius' is something applicable only to the kind of grand mystics and ascetics who have already been dismissed here as either implausible or impractical. Who else but a saint could exercise this kind of moral brilliance? And yet attention itself may give some clues as to the way in which a kind of perfection can be found in the imperfection of juggled life, death, suffering, desires and weaknesses.

It might be too trite and flat to suggest that the lesson of the hawthorn (or cherry) blossom is that death, through its limitation of life, grants life value, but two things should be noted about this trite flatness. Firstly, there is something which must be noted quite pointedly as a key part of the conclusion of this discussion as a whole: that finding the conclusion of a meandering and complex succession of reflections to be very familiar and commonsensical is indicative of true philosophy and precisely what this essay set out to achieve. Secondly: it should be noted that 'trite flatness' is never (and especially when such broad ethical concepts as these are at play) as tritely flat as it seems.

This book began with an exposition of Aristotle's claim that common sense intuitions must play a central role in philosophy as a standard against which theories should be tested. It is worth recalling the passage of the Nicomachean Ethics which was taken as a central tenet of this investigation:

> In matters of emotion and of action, words are less convincing than deeds; when therefore our theories are at variance with palpable facts, they provoke contempt, and involve the truth in their own discredit... Hence it appears that true theories are the most valuable for conduct as well as for science; harmonising with the facts, they carry conviction, and so encourage those who understand them to guide their lives by them.
>
> (Aristotle, *EN*, § X, I; 1172^{a}34–1172^{b}7)

In this way, it is hoped that arriving at an idea of aspects of non-human life being evocative and appropriate sources of inspiration for intuitions which are commonly expressed or held to be true is itself a fitting conclusion for a set of philosophical (or narrative-poetic-participatory-observational) reflections.

As to the matter of these intuitions having greater depth than might at first be apparent, it will be important to return to the manner in which these realisations of value through the apprehension of limitations are 'strangely surprising'.

As aforementioned, careful attention can reveal great importance in that which might otherwise have been dismissed as unimportant. The most peculiar aspect of this suggestion is that it appears at first to fly in the face of an epistemology which sets common intuitions as a primary standard against which reflections, observations and arguments are judged. If on the one hand it is being claimed that things which seem, fairly uncritically, to be correct are indeed correct (or at least are one of the best means at our disposal for judging the accuracy of other suggestions) and on the other hand it is being suggested that the 'unexamined life' is liable to great error, then we may have another contradiction. Yet, it would be a mistake to imagine that the ubiquity and strength of the insights and ways of life against which Aristotle would have us judge our philosophical reflections are synonymous with an uncritical acceptance of all our everyday assumptions and comforts.

First, Aristotle himself is clearly most concerned with practical evidence and the kind of paradoxes with which the Eleatics had played: the fact that multiplicity is observably extant should be given some weight in our thinking. The epistemological tenet with which this discussion began and with which it shall now draw to a close is concerned with significant points of insight and intuition rather than all things which are assumed. It should be recalled that although these two categories may share some grey space they also occupy poles which separate one another to a practical degree. Personal preferences and diverse ways of life will always yield a near infinite array of interpretations as to what is and is not significant in life but even when the bricks and mortar of metaphysical scepticism are discounted, moral questions can still present similarly tangible points of mutual recognition (if not consensus) about which our reflections may turn. Some stories transcend the boundaries of time and place.[15]

Of course, even the most timeless of tales can be the subject of disagreement. Nietzsche finds in Hamlet an ideal of unravelling. Hamlet is witness to the most brutal inconsistencies and injustices of life and through this experience, Nietzsche finds that the prince is liberated from being bound to consistency and justice; he explains that such tragic heroes have:

> ...seen into the essence of things, they have *known*, and it nauseates them to act; since their action can change nothing in the eternal essence of things, they find it laughable or disgraceful that it is expected of them that they reconstruct the world that is out of joint. Knowledge kills action; action requires the veiledness of illusion.
>
> (Nietzsche 1872, p. 40)

And yet others of us would find that Hamlet's lesson in the unfolding of misfortune and injustice is not so much one of inertia and despair (though he may go through a fair bit of this), but rather that through a certain species of incapacity (and, yes, dark melancholy) Hamlet is shocked into seeing a kind of unifying meaning behind the chaos. When he urges Horatio to 'report me and my cause aright' we may question what 'cause' he refers to. Has Hamlet himself not been an agent of entropy, of revenge? Horatio has followed the prince in his quest to bring about the ruin of a king, and we may be reminded of Hamlet's own reflections amidst the graves:

HAMLET
>   To what base uses we may return, Horatio! Why may
>   Not imagination trace the noble dust of Alexander,
>   Till he find it stopping a bung-hole?

HORATIO
>   'Twere to consider too curiously, to consider so.

HAMLET
>   No, faith, not a jot; but to follow him thither with
>   Modesty enough, and likelihood to lead it: as
>   Thus: Alexander died, Alexander was buried,
>   Alexander returneth into dust; the dust is earth; of
>   Earth we make loam; and why of that loam, whereto he
>   Was converted, might they not stop a beer-barrel?
>   Imperious Caesar, dead and turn'd to clay,
>   Might stop a hole to keep the wind away:
>   O, that that earth, which kept the world in awe,
>   Should patch a wall to expel the winter flaw!
>   But soft! but soft! aside: here comes the king (5.1).

Not too curiously, to consider so, not so long as we follow Alexander 'thither with modesty enough, and likelihood to lead it'. Hamlet's impotence becomes intertwined with the impotence of us all; the justice which the prince would exact upon the king is the justice to which all of us, kings too, are subject. Joshua Billings highlights how this kind of 'meaningful' interpretation of Hamlet contrasts with that established by Schopenhauer and Nietzsche (Billings 2012, p. 65). Billings focuses on the way in which the philosophical insights offered by great and timeless drama can be significant points of contention. In reading the more positive conclusions of Walter Benjamin, Billings explains how Hamlet can be understood as exemplifying '...the dialectical worldview of melancholy, in which the mourning and hope are inextricable...' (*Ibid.*, p. 68) and 'As the only figure in whom the gap between consciousness and reflection is bridged, Hamlet redeems baroque eschatology from its tendency to dissolve into meaninglessness' (*Ibid.*, p. 71).

And yet both Nietzsche's reading and readings like those of Benjamin find something powerful and insightful in the prince's meditations on the conflicts and dissolutions of the world. Perhaps even those aspects of our social and moral worlds which seem most secure and universal are susceptible to some kinds of close scrutiny, yet to imagine that this susceptibility renders these hinges incapable of acting as powerful points of reference of the sort Aristotle finds in 'facts' is another thing entirely. These are the great lessons, the great stories; these are the conversations which have always been had and which always must be had as long as philosophy exists. These stories are the grammar of our lives and yet, just because they stand behind everything we think, say and do, it is not true that they are always apparent or heeded.

As common as death and just as surprising.

Grammar, key moral principles, skeletons: unseen yet utterly vital, they form the structure upon which all depends.

Those of us who have cared for those who cannot appreciate this care may know something of this surprise. The elderly, infants, the infirm, non-humans; try cleaning them amidst a torrent of complaint, try healing them only to receive violence, kiss their sleeping brow and marvel at what you find. I have seen these things done without real care and attention; and since I am not a saint and suffer from all the weakness of exhaustion, irritability, pride, indignation, entitlement, impatience, anger and despair, I too have done these things without real care and attention, without love at the centre. I may grow angry at my dog for failing to find a place to defecate swiftly enough in the driving rain, I may despair at a relative who forgets what I have done for them and resent this lack of gratitude, and yet when I do succeed, and when I am able to wade through the filth, the pain and the loneliness, I find that the simplest things constitute a world entire.

When all the screaming has subsided, when all the insults and violence have been endured, when the frozen rain has passed and all that remains are the gleaming drips on the naked branch, then how brilliantly they shine. I may not entirely know if I feel joy or despair but, when I least expect it, the smallest things: a smile, a bound of joy, a brief look of gratitude, a moment of serenity, a green shoot in spring, the wellbeing of another, these little things stand tall as the true home of love. And each time it is strangely surprising. Finding that such small things can outshine the vast darkness, that a simple act of kindness can dwarf all the titanic disjunctions and unthinking chaos of the universe. It doesn't matter how many times this is shown to be true, how many times we forget this lesson and relearn it, this love always comes with a little thrill, a sharp intake of breath as we surface, once again, from the depths of life.

It is the little quirks, faults, foibles, overcoming past traumas, our ability to be the point of strength and comfort for another in a very specific way which reveals love. Paying attention to another helps us see what's loveable. And it is the little details and the grand themes which require this attention. The glaring things which attract or repel require no such time or care, but by giving ourselves into a state of acceptance and understanding, the most precious and fulfilling aspects of shared life can be discovered. The idea that a woodlouse has interests of any particular note may be fanciful to some people, that a tree or even a weed should have capacities to flourish of a similar kind may be equally preposterous yet if we can but spend the time to look and to listen, little worlds open up and reveal continuity between ourselves and life quite generally.

Both universal love, Schweitzer's Christian compassion, and the more proximal and possessive kind of love shine out and grab us like a phoenix from the ashes. It is when we find something broken, something faulty, and we find, in this brokenness, a deeper kind of perfection than we might ever have been able to find in the unblemished version.

The condition of succeeding in balancing the various moral demands which life places on us must be accompanied by (or realised through) a complex kind of attitude which reflects the strangely surprising nature of love uncovered through care and attention.

The Jester's bones

What becomes clear (or as clear as maybe hoped) is that the achievement of this balancing act of wisdom is not borne out in mere equanimity, in emotional and intellectual poise, serenity, or Ἀταραξία, it is, instead, a state of sensitivity, of *'understanding'*; not understanding *of* anything in particular but understanding *as such*: 'understanding' as an adjective rather than a noun or verb: as in 'she is an understanding sort of person', something similar in meaning to 'forgiving' or 'accepting'.

It would be facile to suggest that this wise person, who manages to become familiar with the strangely surprising nature of love and perfection to be found in imperfection, becomes a species of the misty-eyed sea cow, drifting through life with nought but a smug smile to grace their face. This vision of stoic wisdom might be a danger with some models of virtue but this would fail to do justice to the very real magnitude of both the evil and the good which this state of surprise entertains. There are two alternative conditions or attitudes which may offer a more compelling description of wisdom's central attitudes and these are (1) poignancy and (2) good humour.

Poignancy is a good word because it captures the way in which an awareness of flaws can be vital to a sense of value. Poignancy suggests that an awareness of perfection through imperfection necessarily requires that the initial awareness of imperfection is not extinguished by the then coextensive sense of perfection.

When my daughter has given me a scribble of colour on a piece of paper, or a messy clod of soil and grass which she has mangled for me, my description of these gifts as 'perfect' is not quite the same as when I consider the possibility of perfection in *Apollo Belvedere*, nor am I just lying when I say they are perfect; *they are perfect*. Of course, I am not blind to the crudeness and absurd ineptitude of these little offerings. Were I so, then appreciating their perfection would be impossible. It is the achievement of approximation in the face of impossibility which is itself constitutive of the only kind of perfection which is really meaningful. The reason the fragile blossoms are so evocative of wisdom is that they demonstrate the way in which all things are like the least of things. This scribble on this piece of paper is a little piece of generosity, a little piece of playful creation.

My daughter's efforts are demonstrably far from artwork of complete and cosmic perfection, but I don't really know what one of those would be like anyway. I have some sense of the direction in which art must move if it is to better approximate that perfection, but since all such efforts will ulti-mately fail to achieve complete success then each (even those of Leochares or Michelangelo) is akin to my daughter's scribbles, what matters is that they *approximate* perfection.

Mostly, we are blind to these little perfections within imperfection. Impressed by the achievements which seem so much closer to that infinitely distant goal we ignore the little successes all about us. But attention and love can surprise us, they can remind us how small we are and how great every living thing is. And yet, if the brokenness were entirely forgotten, if the small things 'outshone the vast darkness' to the extent that the darkness no longer remained, then these small perfections would cease to be mean-ingful. If the perfection in imperfection were an end, if it were a stopping point, then the virtues would cease to be in motion and cease to resemble perfection in any way; so, it's not *that* kind of perfection. Of Achilles and the tortoise, it is not who arrives at the finish line which is most interesting, but that they are both moving towards it.

Dewi Phillips judged I. T. Ramsey harshly for his employment of Kierkegaard's 'infinite approximation' (Phillips 1976, pp. 477–487). In *Religious Language,* Ramsey seeks to use the Eleatic-esque mathematical analogy of an infinite series leading to a point to suggest how increments of moral superiority can demonstrate the divine perfection which they approx-imate. In this way particular good lives, for all their faults, converging at an infinitely distant point of perfection, permit a certain kind of knowl-edge of God (Ramsey 1957). Phillips is convinced that Ramsey has things backwards; it is the series itself which depends first on the notion of God which Ramsey employs rather than the series which offers knowledge of God (Phillips 1976, p. 484). What is more, Phillips contends, there are clear examples of moral questions where this kind of linear scale of goodness is simply not applicable, cases, for example, where everyone is at fault (*Ibid.*, p. 485). As previously in this discussion, those figures who's thought is most crucial to my own are those with whom I must both agree and disagree; Phillips is no exception.

If Ramsey spoke instead, rather than of 'God', of 'The Good' or 'Goodness', would Phillips have less to complain about? If the ideal moral perfection at which these fine examples (never) converged were a less religiously loaded idea, then would this infinite approximation make sense? Phillips suggests that disagreement about what kinds of examples of moral behaviour should be counted and how they should be prioritised would still mean that any such series of better or worse moral examples could never be truly meaningful. Yet, if Phillips' suggestion that Ramsey's idea of God is logically prior to his series were agreed upon, and 'Goodness' (the possibility of being better or worse as such) were substituted for 'God' then should this pluralism argument hold any sway? As has been suggested, the idea that more extreme examples of virtue and vice could not provide at least a starting point for this kind of discussion seems at least a bit disingenuous if not entirely dishonest. Indeed, this is precisely the reason this book began with an exposition of a certain kind of moral realism because it is the concession of the reality of this kind of 'goodness as such' which acts as a precondition of wrestling with the fractured and occasionally oppositional activity of juggling the virtues (and conceiving of ourselves as being better or worse: morally improving). So Phillips appears to be quite right to suggest that Ramsey is going at things back-to-front, but if we are not looking for proof of God (or goodness) but instead just for a good way to think about our own moral improvement (or deterioration) and thereby improve more effectively, could Ramsey's model of infinite approximation still be of use?

It is with Phillips' ultimate objection to Ramsey that this book finds greatest concordance. Phillips suggests that the very idea of divine perfection makes nonsense of the goodness(es) we find in this imperfect world, the idea of our goods being devoid of their imperfections sterilises and nullifies their meaning (*Ibid.*, pp. 485–486). By way of illustration Phillips turns to Wallace Stevens' poem *Sunday Morning* and it is worth repeating the sixth stanza here:

> Is there no change of death in paradise?
> Does ripe fruit never fall? Or do the boughs
> Hang always heavy in that perfect sky,
> Unchanging, yet so like our perishing earth,
> With rivers like our own that seek for seas
> They never find, the same receding shores
> That never touch with inarticulate pang?
> Why set the pear upon those river-banks
> Or spice the shores with odors of the plum?
> Alas, that they should wear our colors there,
> The silken weavings of our afternoons,
> And pick the strings of our insipid lutes!
> Death is the mother of beauty, mystical,
> Within whose burning bosom we devise
> Our earthly mothers waiting, sleeplessly.

(Stevens 1967, p. 33)

And perhaps there is just some confusion about the idea of perfection here. Maybe Ramsey's mistake was in discussing the perfection of God as opposed to another kind of perfection. It would seem entirely plausible to suggest that 'perfection' could just mean something beyond which we cannot meaningfully or conscionably desire. And it would seem implausible for Phillips to object to an approximation of this kind of perfection. Perfection could be imagined as the opposite of imperfection or it could be imagined as that in which we should rejoice and which we should find fulfilling.

It may well be suggested that as soon as perfection loses its mystical sense of incomprehensibility and enters the realms of 'just something beyond which we cannot meaningfully or conscionably desire', then a qualitative line has been crossed which alters the idea beyond recognition. If the kind of perfection being talked about is not faultlessness and is just a sense of contentment with one's lot and acceptance of the faults of loved ones, then the idea of approximation is unnecessary. Far from being approximated, this kind of perfection is regularly achieved and is conceptually unproblematic. When a 'wise' person manages to achieve a reasonable balance of courage, cleverness, compassion, justice, personal love, aesthetic appreciation, patience, attention etc., then we could just say that they have achieved a kind of goodness beyond which we cannot reasonably expect anyone to go.

It would, though, be absurd to suggest that imperfection is desirable if one meant by imperfection things which are undesirable, such a flat contradiction would be beyond even the permissions of this discussion's relaxed epistemology. What may not, however, be a flat contradiction, is the suggestion that imperfection does consist of all those sorts of things which possess undesirable elements but without which we cannot conceive of a world which is better than this.

Killing is, in relative isolation, bad. I can see the fear and hear the pain, it is horrific. I can, just about, paint crude fictions in which killing doesn't happen and these visions (for all the details they neglect) are pleasant things. There is a sense in which less killing draws towards an ideal of no killing, a perfect, non-violent world. Denying members of my family (human or non-human) freedoms and pleasures is, in relative isolation, bad. I can, again, paint crude pictures of worlds in which all of their desires are fulfilled, all of their needs met and there is no cause to restrain or chastise. The reason that these fantasy worlds, so incompatible in their respective content, are so similar, is that they draw on a common principle of improvement, to deny them an orientation towards improvement, towards perfection, would render them as meaningless as these two-dimensional images would render the whole.

The infinite approximation which can escape Phillips' objections is ultimately a kind of dynamic compromise. This approximation needn't always be linear and perhaps Phillips is right about the implausibility of such a scale, but this need not mean that a constant attempt to balance all moral demands is meaningless. It is the constant need to pay attention, to assess, to judge and act accordingly in perpetually shifting circumstances which gives wisdom the peculiar quality of simultaneous tension and ease which is expressed in the attitude of poignancy.

Regret and contentment, sadness and joy, action and acceptance. The attitude is itself a psychological manifestation of the balance and compromise achieved in moral learning.

And yet, there is something missing. All of this oh-so-worthy sense of poignancy or pathos is just a bit dour. Wallace Stevens' poem rings very true and is wonderfully evocative of the sense of intermingled darkness and light which lies at the heart of this theory of wisdom, but his 'insipid lutes' and 'silken weavings' just seem a bit clean. The 'tears of things' so far seem to be very heavy tears, very serious. I, for one, in reading Stevens' poem, cannot help but hear, amidst all the languid serenity of this scene, a tuneful and unexpected little fart.

Flatulence is a wonderful thing for informing humility. The moving magnificence of the natural world which can be witnessed in the garden, all dappled sunlight and mossy skeletons, can draw one into a sense of grand and cosmic significance: an Apollonian reverie full of the promise of insight and philosophy. This dream is disrupted brilliantly by the improbably long farts of an unseen horse. The little fragile things of life aren't just pathetic, they aren't just models of the universe in microcosm, they are funny.

The 'strangely surprising' nature of the realisations at the heart of wisdom share much in common with jokes. The idea that great facades crumble to nought is not just expressive of poignancy, it is also a bit ridiculous. The near contradictory nature of finding perfection in imperfection, of finding greatness in the little things, has similarities with incongruity theories of humour.[16] When something unexpected happens which contrasts in an ironic sort of way with that which preceded it, this is funny.

There's nothing wiser than a joke at a funeral. They call it 'gallows humour' sometimes but that can carry a sense of desperate ignorance, of looking the other way, and of dishonesty. Undoubtedly there are jokes which can act in this way, to draw attention away from dreadful things, but there are jokes at funerals which are not like this at all. Very great and weighty matters, particularly the death of a loved one, can become overwhelming and threaten to engulf us in despair by obscuring less conspicuous details. Incongruity is like a slap in the face, undignified and base realities can cure us of a false sense of magnitude and importance, they can help us gain a sense of perspective. When we talk about that time when she became hopelessly drunk and vomited on his lap, or when, as a child, he groped the breasts of someone he shouldn't. These kinds of memories can act as a way of realigning our attention away from just the utter limit of life and its greatest heights, back to the person as a whole, warts and all.

And how you miss every blemish of his skin, his bad breath and just the way he wagged his tail. Those absurd little things.

And we will laugh with a splutter through the snot as it rolls down our lips, mixing with the tears.

Wisdom is the act of not giving up that snot-soaked laugh, not forgetting it or discarding it as soon as the passions have passed, but instead holding it there behind a more sustainable, everyday approach to life. This is the 'smile' which has been repeated throughout this book, it is the attitude of a man accused by his peers of corrupting the young, of not taking himself or others too seriously.

Permaculture acts as a constant reminder of the absurd little things. The stupid antics of the dogs and the pigs are a wonderful counterpoint to the enormity of death, of wars and disease. Crushing cabbage white caterpillars between my fingers is a grim business, but it is done amidst the brilliant hues of the delicate nasturtiums, and still, the ravens will twist and play and giggle. Perhaps this laughter dances dangerously close to a precipice of madness, and this may present a concession to Chesterton's fears and the risks Strawson finds in narrative life. Wisdom undoubtedly resides in the ability to balance a range of seemingly incompatible qualities, to carry as great a weight of learning, detail and responsibility as one is able, so perhaps there is a sense in which this weight pushes a mind to the brink of insanity, but certainly not beyond.

The breadth of wisdom is itself a guard against insanity, it is a kind of moral and psychological spreading of risk; one is less likely to find oneself suddenly overwhelmed and broken by an unforeseen moral dilemma if a very great range of moral dilemmas, the manifold depths, darknesses and triumphs of life have already been foreseen. Of course, there is a fine line between spreading risk and overstretching supply lines but the two are not mutually exclusive. Philosophy, through this spreading of risk, once again aligns with permaculture; it returns to basic facts, to the fundamental elements of which our lives are composed, in order to build a robust basis for life. And what is exposed through symbiotic ethics is the way in which actually doing permaculture can itself be a kind of pre-cerebral philosophy, it's practical mirroring of the principles of philosophy becomes a physical medium by which the ethos of loving wisdom can be learned. As an Aristotelean training in virtue, permaculture can come to instil a deep sense of the importance of fundamental things, of basic things, of honest things. But it is not all roses, it is also a lesson in the closeness of beauty to darkness, of death to life, of joy to pain.

And so, once again, we have returned to a balancing act. When we live amidst life, between the demands of logic and the pressures of common sense, along the intangible tightrope of aesthetic cohesion and moral intuition, between a desire for knowledge and an acceptance of our own limitations, between Scylla and Charybdis, amongst the whirling and swirling and screaming and laughing and eating and scratching and crying and dying of δαίμων, we need a friend. Wisdom is our friend, our ally, and we must be an ally to wisdom. Wisdom is exactly this balancing act and it is formed and bolstered by all of these little opportunities to exercise virtue.

This book has attempted to offer a theory of wisdom, a picture of what wisdom might be like and how it might be found amongst the worms. Perhaps this picture will remain incomplete if it is not also accompanied by the practical exercise of attempting some actual symbiotic ethics, or even some permaculture; perhaps there is an inherent contradiction in writing a book about how philosophy cannot be done simply by writing books. It should, I think, at the very least, include an explicit recommendation to grow a vegetable. I do that now.

Grow a vegetable.

If any of my musings and rambling, woolly pseudo-arguments have rung hollow then try it. If you do not already do so, then plant a vegetable seed in some soil, help it to grow, and then eat the vegetable. If you already do this then well done, I salute you, you're half-way there.

But remember how difficult it all is, don't expect a simple answer, don't expect a miracle solution, because there's no such thing. Whilst it all might point in the same direction, towards goodness, truth and beauty, the pieces will never fit together perfectly, and if you ever think you've reached the end then you will have failed, you will have walked away from life. Stay with it; stay close, yet not too close, tread that fine line which demands constant reassessment, constant self-assessment, constant attention. And if you can do this constant thing then you will be a bit more than half-way there, you will be a friend to wisdom, a philosopher, closest to the gods.

Notes

1 It is fair to say that Cooper acknowledges this phenomenon of the garden as art and he is chiefly concerned with this as a virtuous practice. This is just a different approach and since there is some convergence with Cooper in the aesthetic approach of this book there is room to think that these two approaches might find some synthesis or overlap (Cooper 2006, pp. 21–61).

2 Of course, at its mid-century inception, 'back-to-the-land' often represented a wholesale attempt to escape 'wage slavery' entirely as Dona Brown (2011, p. 211) notes in *Back to the Land: The Enduring Dream of Self-Sufficiency in Modern America*.

3 Which is to say, Stoicism.

4 *Cf.* J. Malpas and R. C. Solomon, 'Introduction' to J. Malpas and R. C. Solomon (Ed.), *Philosophy and Death*, (London, Routledge, 1998), p. 1.

5 As aforementioned, these associations come in differing degrees of frequency. Old age and wisdom are certainly a common pairing (a discussion of wider important and extensive history which can only be touched upon here). The Association between old age and gardening has far more to do with wage-based economics and traditions of retirement and, as such, is (thankfully) restricted to a more narrow selection of humanity. These cultural associations of gardening in a British context are explored in greater detail by Lisa Taylor (2008, p. 112) in *A Taste for Gardening: Classed and Gendered Practices*.

6 I am talking specifically about 'earthworms' of the order Ogligochaeta of which there are over 5000 recognised species, see C. A. Edwards and P. J.

Bohlen's (1977, pp. 114–115) *Biology and Ecology of Earthworms*. On the significance of this group of animals it is worth noting Charles Darwin's remark that 'It may be doubted whether there are many other animals which have played so important a part in the history of the world, as have these lowly organized creatures' (Darwin 1904, p. 288).

7 For an example where this association has reached the point of being a simple translation, see de Angelis' (2012, p. 19) *The Japanese Effect in Contemporary Irish Poetry*.

8 David Wharton (2008, p. 276) has offered a gratifyingly rigorous analysis of this half-line of Virgil's epic (which has achieved a level of ubiquity that makes taking its meaning for granted a real risk) *in Sunt Lacrimae Rerum: An Exploration in Meaning*. Here Wharton takes the view that the ambiguity of the phrase serves to interrupt the reader and give them pause for thought. I am inclined to agree (I should like to agree) with Wharton that this sort of technique fits well with the elegance and subtlety of Virgil's work but I would also add that this kind of interruption fits both the mood of the sentiment itself and its setting. Aeneas is engaged in an interruption of his journey, he must stop and think and the awkwardness and possible expansiveness of this phrase lends a certain weight to its probable philosophical content in the shape of the concepts and virtues discussed here (from patience to poignancy).

9 Steve Odin (2016, pp. 275–276) gives a good summary of the way in which both 'mono no aware' and 'aware' as such are subject to a complex ongoing discussion as to how these terms should be understood.

10 Douglas Cairns (2014, p. 107) draws a connection between ancient Greek senses of this transitoriness reflected in literature and the Japanese tradition in *Exemplarity and Narrative in the Greek Tradition*.

11 On the central place of Sakura Zensen (1998, pp. 213–236) (the 'Cherry Blossom Front' which moves across Japan as the spring progresses), see E. Ohnuki-Tierney's *Cherry Blossoms and Their Viewing: A Window onto Japanese Culture*.

12 As is noted by Richard Maybe (1996, p. 212) in *Flora Britannica*.

13 On these associations see M. Inaba and Y. Inaba's (1992, p. 93) *Human Body Odor: Etiology, Treatment and Related Factors*.

14 Again noted by Maybe (1996, p. 212).

15 E. M. Forster goes so far as to imagine all storytellers ('English novelists') sitting in a transcendent room together (as if it were in a Platonic realm of Forms); 'History develops, art stands still' (Forster 1927, p. 27).

16 On an incongruity theory of humour see N. Carroll's (2014, pp. 49–50) *Humour: A Very Short Introduction*. No further exposition will be offered here of theories of humour, not only for the reason that these are unnecessary for the points being made here but also because attempting to reduce humour to a set of causes or conditions risks a kind of inappropriate reductionism. It is tempting to wheel Bernard Williams back out for the sake of defending the suggestion that asking *why* something is funny is just 'one thought too many'; ask that kind of question and it might just stop being funny.

Bibliography

Ackah, E. K. 2003, 'Socratic Wisdom', in *History of Philosophy Quarterly*, vol. 20, no. 2, pp. 123–147.

Adams, D. 1982, *Life, the Universe and Everything*, London: Macmillan, 2010.

_____. 1984, *So Long and Thanks for All the Fish*, London: Pan Books, 2009.

de Angelis, I. 2012, *The Japanese Effect in Contemporary Irish Poetry*, Houndmills: Palgrave Macmillan.

Anscombe, G. E. M. 1958, 'Modern Moral Philosophy', in *Philsosophy*, vol. 33, no. 124, pp. 1–19.

_____. 1957, *Intention*, Ithaca, NY: Cornell University Press, 1968.

Ansell-Pearson, K. 1992, 'Who Is the Ubermensch? Time, Truth, and Woman in Nietzsche', *Journal of the History of Ideas*, vol. 53, no. 2, pp. 309–331.

Aristotle. 1933, *Metaphysics*, Tedennick, H. (tr.), Cambridge, MA: Harvard University Press.

_____. 1934, *Nicomachean Ethics*, Rackham, H. (tr.), Cambridge, MA: Harvard University Press.

_____. 1957, *Politics*, Ross, W. D. (tr./ed.), Oxford: Clarendon Press.

_____. 1957, *De Anima*, London: Harvard University Press.

_____. 1995, 'On the Soul', Smith, J. A. (tr.), in Barnes, J. (ed.), *The Complete Works of Aristotle*: The Revised Oxford Translation, Vol. 1, Chichester: Princeton University Press.

_____ 1995, 'Posterior Analytics', Barnes, J. (tr.), in Barnes, J. (ed.),*The Complete Works of Aristotle*, Princeton, NJ: Princeton University Press, pp. 114–166.

_____. 1995, 'Politics', Jowett, B. (tr.), in Barnes, J. (ed.),*The Complete Works of Aristotle: The Revised Oxford Translation*, Vol. 2, Chichester: Princeton University Press, pp. 1986–2129.

Assmann, J. 2012, 'Cultural Memory and the Myth of the Axial Age', in Bellah, R. N. and Joas, H. (eds.), *The Axial Age and Its Consequences*, Cambridge, MA: Belknap. pp. 366–409.

Athanassoulis, N. 2014, 'Educating for Virtue', in van Hooft, S. (ed.), *The Handbook of Virtue Ethics*, Oxford: Routledge, pp. 440–450.

Bacchini, F., Caputo, S. and Dell'Utri, M. 2014, *Metaphysics and Ontology Without Myths*, Newcastle: Cambridge Scholars.

Bacharach, S. and Harold, J. 2015, 'Aesthetic and Artistic Value', in Ribeiro, A. C. (ed.), *The Bloomsbury Companion to Aesthetics*, London: Bloomsbury.

Benson, H. H. 2000, *Socratic Wisdom: The Model of Knowledge in Plato's Early Dialogues*, Oxford: Oxford University Press.

Bentham, J. 1780, *An Introduction to the Principles of Morals and Legislation*, Oxford: Clarendon Press, 1996.

Barfield, R. 2011, *The Ancient Quarrel Between Philosophy and Poetry*, Cambridge: Cambridge University Press.

Billings, J. 2012, 'Spectres of *Hamlet* in Benjamin and the German Theory of Tragedy' in Owen, R. J. (ed.), *The Hamlet Zone: Reworking Hamlet for European Cultures*, Newcastle upon Tyne: Cambridge Scholars Publishing, 2012.

Billing, M. 2013, *Learn to Write Badly: How to Succeed in the Social Sciences*, Cambridge: Cambridge University Press.

Blondell, R. 2004, *The Play of Character in Plato's Dialogues*, Cambridge: Cambridge University Press.

Bobzien, S. 2000, 'Did Epicurus Discover the Free Will Problem?', in *Oxford Studies in Ancient Philosophy*, Vol. XIX, pp. 286–337.

Brandon, W. P. 1982, '"Fact" and "Value" in the Thought of Peter Winch: Linguistic Analysis Broaches Metaphysical Questions', in *Political Theory*, vol. 10, no. 2, pp. 215–244.

Brickhouse, T. C. and Smith, N. D. 1997, 'Socrates and the Unity of the Virtues', *The Journal of Ethics*, vol. 1, no. 4, pp. 311–324.

Brown, D. 2011, *Back to the Land: The Enduring Dream of Self-Sufficiency in Modern America*, London: The University of Wisconsin Press.

Brown, M. F. 2008, 'Cultural Relativism 2.0.', *Current Anthropology*, vol. 49, no. 3, pp. 363–383.

Brukamp, K. 2000, 'Elements of Eudaemonia: Capabilities and Functionings' in Kallhoff, A. (ed.), *Martha C. Nussbaum: Ethics and Political Philosophy*, London: Transaction Publishers, pp. 93–104.

Bugos, P. E. and McCarthy, L. M. 1984, 'Ayoreo Infanticide: A Case Study', in Hausfater, G. and Hardy, S. B. (eds.), *Infanticide: Comparative and Evolutionary Perspectives*, Aldine: New York, pp. 503–520.

Burbules, N. C. and Smeyers, P. 2003, 'Wittgenstein, the Practice of Ethics, and Moral Education', in Fletcher, S. (ed.), *Philosophy of Education*, Vol. 2002, Urbana, IL: Philosophy of Education Society, pp. 248–257.

Burch, R. 2002, 'Thinking Between Philosophy and Poetry', in Verdicchio, M. and Burch, R. (eds.), *Between Philosophy and Poetry*, London: Continuum.

Cairns, D. 2014, 'Exemplarity and Narrative in the Greek Tradition', in Cairns, D. and Scodel, R. (eds.), *Defining Greek Narrative*, Edinburgh: Edinburgh University Press.

Capra, F. and Luisi, P. L. 2014, *The Systems View of Life: A Unifying Vision*, Cambridge: Cambridge University Press.

Carroll, N. 2014, *Humour: A Very Short Introduction*, Oxford: Oxford University Press.

Case, T. 1925, 'The Development of Aristotle', in *Mind*, New Series, vol. 34, no. 133, pp. 80–86.

Chesterton, G. K. 1908, *Orthodoxy*, London: John Lane The Bodley Head, 1943.

Clough, D. L. 2012, *On Animals: Volume One, Systematic Theology*, London: Bloomsbury.

Cockburn, D. 1994, 'Human Beings and Giant Squids', *Philosophy*, vol. 69, no. 268, pp. 135–150.

———. 1990, *Other Human Beings*, London: Macmillan.

Cooper, D. 2006, *A Philosophy of Gardens*, Oxford: Oxford University Press.

Cooper, J. M. 1985, 'Aristotle on the Goods of Fortune', *The Philosophical Review*, vol. 94, no. 2, pp. 173–196.

_____. 2013, *Pursuits of Wisdom*, Oxford: Princeton University Press.

Copleston, F. 1947, *A History of Philosophy*, Vol. 1, Norwich: Burns, Oates and Washbourne.

Cutler, I. 2005, *Cynicism from Diogenes to Dilbert*, Jefferson, NC: McFarland.

Darcus, S. 1974, '"Daimon" as a Force Shaping "Ethos' in Heraclytus', *Phoenix*, vol. 28, no. 4, pp. 390–407.

Darwin, C. 1904, *The Formation of Vegetable Mould Through the Action of Worms*, London: John Murray.

Davies, W. H. 1911, 'Leisure', in *Songs of Joy and Others*, London: Fifield.

De La Bellacasa, M. 2017, *Matters of Care: Speculative Ethics in More than Human Worlds*, London: University of Minnesota Press.

Demetrius of Phalerum. 1902, *De Elocutione*, Roberts W. R. (ed.), Cambridge: Cambridge University Press.

den Otter, A. A. 2012, *Civilising the Wilderness*, Edmonton: University of Alberta Press.

Devettere, R. J. 2002, *Introduction to Virtue Ethics: Insights of the Ancient Greeks*, Washington, DC: Georgetown University Press.

Dobson, A. et al. 2008, 'Homage to Linnaeus: How Many Parasites? How Many Hosts?', in *Proceedings of the National Academy of Sciences of the United States of America*, vol. 105, no. Supplement 1.

Don, M. 2016, 'The Full Monty', BBC Gardeners', World Magazine, August.

Duderstadt, J. J. 2000, *A University for the 21st Century*, Ann Arbour, MI: University of Michigan Press.

Edwards, C. A. and Bohlen, P. J. 1977, *Biology and Ecology of Earthworms*, London: Chapman and Hall.

Empiricus, S. 1933, *Outlines of Pyrrhonism*, Bury, R. G. (tr.), Cambridge, MA: Harvard University Press.

Ettema, J. S. and Glasser, T. L. 1990, Narrative Form and Moral Force: The Realization of Innocence and Guilt Through Investigative Journalism', in Brock, B., Scott, L. and Chesebro, L. (eds.), *Methods of Rhetorical Criticism*, Detroit, MI: Wayne State University Press.

Favela, L. H. and Chemero, A. 2016, 'The Animal-Environment System', in Coello, Y. and Fischer, M. H. (eds.), *Perceptual and Emotional Embodiment: Foundations of Embodied Cognition*, Vol. 1, Oxford: Routledge, pp. 59–74.

Fischer, J. M. and Ravizza, M. (ed.). 1993, *Perspectives on Moral Responsibility*, London: Cornell University Press, pp. 1–44.

Fisher, W. R. 1990, 'The Narrative Paradigm: An Elaboration', in Brock, B. L., Scott, R. L. and Chesebro, J. W. (eds.), *Methods of Rhetorical Criticism*, Detroit, MI: Wayne State University Press.

Forster, E. M. 1927, *Aspects of the Novel*, London: Penguin.

Fox, K. 2013, 'Putting Permaculture Ethics to Work: Commons Thinking, Progress, and Hope', in Lockyer, J. and Veteto, J. R. (eds.), *Environmental Anthropology Engaging Ecotopia: Bioregionalism, Permaculture, and Ecovillages*, Oxford: Berghahn, pp. 164–179.

Francione, G. L. 2010, 'The Abolition of Animal Exploitation', in Francione, G. L. and Garner, R. (eds.), *The Animal Rights Debate: Abolition or Regulation?*, New York, NY: Columbia University Press.

Frankfurt, H. G. 2004, *The Reasons of Love*, Oxford: Princeton University Press.

_____. 1971, 'Freedom of the Will and the Concept of a Person', *The Journal of Philosophy*, vol. 68, no. 1, pp. 5–20.

_____. 1969, 'Alternate Possibilities and Moral Responsibility', *The Journal of Philosophy*, vol. 66, no. 23, pp. 829–839.

Frazer, J. G. 1890, *The Golden Bough: A Study in Magic and Religion*, Fraser, R. (ed.), Oxford: Oxford University Press, 1998.

Frey, R. G. 2011, 'Utilitarianism and Animals', in Beuachamp, T. L. and Frey, R. G. (eds.), *The Oxford Handbook of Animal Ethics*, Oxford: Oxford University Press, pp. 172–193.

Fukuoka, M. 1978, *One Straw Revolution*, Korn, L. (tr.), New York, NY: New York Review Books, 2009.

Gaita, R. 2003, *The Philosopher's Dog*, London: Routledge.

Gandhi, M. K. 1951, *Non-Violent Resistance (Satyagraha)*, Kumarappa, B. (eds.), New York, NY: Shocken Books, 1961 (compiled 1951).

Gardner, H. 1993, *Multiple Intelligences: New Horizons*, New York, NY: Basic Books, 2006.

Gaut, B. 2001, "The Ethical Criticism of Art', in Levinson, J. (ed.), *Aesthetics and Ethics*, Cambridge: Cambridge University Press.

Geertz, C. 1974, 'From the Native's Point of View: On the Nature of Anthropological Understanding', *Bulletin of the American Academy of Arts and Sciences*, vol. 28, no. 1, pp. 26–45.

_____. 1973, *The Interpretation of Cultures*, New York, NY: Basic Book.

Gertler, B. 2005, 'In Defense of Mind-Body Dualism', in Feinberg, J. and Shafer-Landau, R. (eds.), *Reason and Responsibility*, Belmont, CA: Thomson Wadsworth, pp. 285–298.

Gill, J. H. 1982, 'Winch Science and Embodiment', *Soundings: An Interdisciplinary Journal*, vol. 65, no. 4, pp. 417–429.

Goodheart, E. 2009, *Darwinian Misadventures in the Humanities*, London: Transaction.

Griffin, N. 2004, 'The Prehistory of Russell's Paradox', in Link, G. (ed.), *One Hundred Years Of Russell's Paradox*, New York, NY: Walter de Gruyter, pp. 349–372.

Gross, R. 2010, *Psychology: The Science of Mind and Behaviour*, 6th edition, Oxford: Hodder.

Hadot, P. 1995, *What Is Ancient Philosophy*, Chase, M. (tr.), London: Harvard University Press, 2002.

_____. 1987, *Philosophy as a Way of Life*, Chase, M. (tr.), Oxford: Blackwell, 1995.

Hauskeller, M. 2002, 'The Relation Between Ethics and Aesthetics in Connection with Moral Judgements about Gene Technology', in Heaf, D. and Wirz, J. (eds.), *Genetic Engineering and the Intrinsic Value and Integrity of Animals and Plants*, International Forum for Genetic Engineering, Hafan: Llanystumdwy, pp. 99–102.

Heartshorne, C. and Peden, C. 2010, *Whitehead's View of Reality*, Newcastle: Cambridge Scholars.

Hegel, G. W. F. 1807, *Phenomenology of Spirit*, Miller, A. V. (tr.), Oxford: Oxford University Press.

Heidegger, M. 1946, 'Letter on "Humanism"', in McNeill, W. (tr./ed.), *Pathmarks*, Cambridge: Cambridge University press, 1999.

_____. 1927, *Being and Time*, Mcaquarrie, J. and Robinson, E. (trs.), Oxford: Blackwell, 2001.

Hume, D. 1748, *An Enquiry Concerning Human Understanding*, Oxford: Oxford University Press, 2008.

Hurn, S. 2012, *Humans and Other Animals: Cross Cultural Perspectives on Human-Animal Interactions*, London: Pluto Press.

Hutto, D. 2003, *Wittgenstein and the End of Philosophy: Neither Theory nor Therapy*, Houndmills: Palgrave Macmillan.

Inaba, M. and Inaba, Y. 1992, *Human Body Odor: Etiology, Treatment and Related Factors*, Tokyo: Springer.

Ingold, T. 2014, 'That's Enough About Ethnography', *Hau: Journal of Ethnographic Theory*, vol. 4, no. 1, pp. 383–395.

_____. 2000, *The Perception of The Environment*, London: Routledge.

Issa, K. 1996, 'Untitled (Sakura/Death)', in Bowers, F. (tr./ed.),*The Classic Tradition of Haiku*, New York, NY: Dover.

James, W. 1907, *Pragmatism*, Cambridge: Hackett, 1981.

Johnson, D., Allison, C. and Baron-Cohen, S. 2013, 'The Prevalence of Synesthesia: The Consistency of Revolution', in Simner, J. and Hubbard, E. M. (eds.), *The Oxford Handbook of Synesthesia*, Oxford: Oxford University Press, pp. 3–22.

Joy, M. 2009, 'In Search of Wisdom', in Cornwell, J. and McGhee, M. (eds.), *Philosophers and God: At the Frontiers of Faith and Reason*, London: Continuum.

Kant, I. 1873, *Fundamental Principles of the Metaphysics of Morals*, Kingsmill Abbot, T. (tr.), New York, NY: Cosimo Classics, 2008.

Keenan, J. F. 1996, 'Dualism in Medicine, Christian Theology, and the Aging', *Journal of Religion and Health*, Vol. 35, no. 1, pp. 33–45.

Kenny, A. 2010, *History of Western Philosophy*, Oxford: Oxford University Press.

Kipling, R. 1910, *If*, London: O'Mara, 2016.

Krell, D. F. 1987, 'Daimon Life, Nearness and Abyss: An Introduction to Za-Ology.', *Research in Phenomenology*, vol. 17, pp. 23–53.

Korn, L. 2015, *One Straw Revolutionary: The Philosophy and Work of Masanobu Fukuoka*, White River Junction, VT: Chelsea Green Publishing.

Lafolette, H. and Shanks, N. 1996, 'The Origin of Speciesism', *Philosophy*, vol. 71, pp. 41–61.

Lampert, K. 2013, *Meritocratic Education and Social Worthlessness*, Houndmills: Palgrve Macmillan.

Lango, J. W. 2001, 'Does Whitehead's Metaphysics Contain an Ethics', *Transactions of the Charles S. Peirce Society*, vol. 37, no. 4, pp. 515–536.

LeBon, T. 2001, *Wise Therapy*, London: Continuum.

Lewis, C. S. 1960, *The Four Loves*, London: Harper Collins, 2002.

_____. 1958, 'Religion and Rocketry', in Walmsley, L. (ed.), *C. S. Lewis: Essay Collection and Other Short Pieces*, London: Harper Collins, 2000, pp. 231–236.

Livingstone Smith, D. 2011, *Less Than Human: Why We Demean, Enslave, and Exterminate Others*, New York, NY: Macmillan.

Lobetti, T. F. 2014, *Ascetic Practicses in Japanese Religion*, Oxford: Routledge.

MacIntyre, A. 1981, 'The Nature of Virtues', in Sterba, J. P. (ed.), *Ethics: The Big Questions*, Oxford: Blackwell, 1998, pp. 277–291.

MacIntyre, A. and Bell, D. R. 1967, 'The Idea of a Social Science', *Proceedings of the Aristotelian Society, Supplementary Volumes*, vol. 41, pp. 95–132.

McCarthy, E. 2011, 'Beyond the Binary: Watsuji Tetsuro and Luce Irigaray on Body, Self and Ethics', in Davis, B. W., Schroeder, B. and Wirth, J. M. (eds.), *Japanese and Continental Philosophy*, Bloomington, IN: Indiana University Press.

McCutcheon, R. T. 2005, 'The Autonomy of Religious Experience (Introduction)', in McCutcheon, R. T. (ed.), *The Insider/Outsider Problem in the Study of Religion*, London: Bloomsbury, pp. 67–73.

Malpas, J. and Solomon, R. C. 1998, 'Introduction', in Malpas, J. and Solomon, R. C. (eds.), *Philosophy and Death*, London: Routledge, 1998.

Aurelius, M. 1930, *Mediatations*, Haines, C. R. (tr.), *London*: Harvard University Press.

Marques, A. 2010, 'Anthropological Representations and Forms of Life in Wittgenstein', in Galvez, J. P. (ed.), *Philosophical Anthropology*, Lancaster: Gazelle Books, pp. 61–72.

Martin, M. W. 2007, *Albert Schweitzer's Reverence for Life*, Aldershot: Ashgate.

Maybe, R. 1996, *Flora Britannica*, London: Chatto and Windus.

Midgley, M. 1983, *Animals and Why They Matter*, Athens, GA: University of Georgia Press, 1998.

de Montaigne, M. 1580, 'That to Philosophise Is to Learn How to Die', Florio, J. (tr.), in de Montaigne, M. (ed.), *Montaigne's Essays*, London: The Folio Society, 2006, pp. 61–80.

Monk, R. 1990, *Ludwig Wittgenstein: The Duty of Genius*, London: Random House.

Muelder Eaton, M. 2001, *Merit, Aesthetic and Ethical*, Oxford: Oxford University Press.

Murdoch, I. 1970, *The Sovereignty of Good*, London: Routledge, 1974.

Nabokov, V. 1955, 'Lolita', in *Collins Collectors Choice: Vladimir Nabokov*, London: Collins, 1971.

Nagarjuna. 1995, *Mulamadhyamakakarika (The Fundamental Wisdom of the Middle Way)*, Garfield, J. L. (tr.), Oxford: Oxford University Press.

Ngai, P. 2016, 'Incomplete Subjects: Circular Migration and the Life and Death Struggles of the Migrant Workers in China', in Solé, C., Parella, S., Sordé Martí, T. and Nita, S. (eds.), *Impact of Circular Migration on Human, Political and Civil Rights*, London: Springer, pp. 175–194.

Nehamas, A. 2001, 'H. H. Benson, Socratic Wisdom: The Model of Knowledge in Plato's Early Dialogues, Review' in *Mind*, New Series, vol. 110, no. 439, pp. 717–721.

Nietzsche, F. 1886, 'Beyond Good and Evil', Zimmem, H. and Cohn, P. V. (trs.), in Nietzsche, F. (ed.), *Human All Too Human and Beyond Good and Evil*, Ware: Wordsworth Editions, 2008, pp. 513–690.

_____. 1872, *The Birth of Tragedy and Other Writings*, Geuss, R. (ed.) and Speirs, R. (tr./ed.), Cambridge: Cambridge University Press, 2000.

Noë, R. A. 1994, 'Wittgenstein, Phenomenology and What It Makes Sense to Say.', *Philosophy and Phenomenological Research*, vol. 54, no. 1, pp. 1–42.

Nussbaum, M. C. 2011, *Creating Capabilities*, London: Harvard University Press.

_____. 1994, *Therapy of Desire: Theory and Practice in Hellenistic Ethics*, Oxford: Princeton University Press, 2004.

_____. 1998, 'Non-Relative Virtues', in Sterba, J. P. (ed.), *Ethics: The Big Questions*, Oxford: Blackwell, pp. 259–276.

Odin, S. 2016, *Tragic Beauty in Whitehead and Japanese Aesthetics*, London: Lexington.

Ohnuki-Tierney, E. 1998, 'Cherry Blossoms and Their Viewing: A Window onto Japanese Culture', in Linhart, S. and Früstück, S. (eds.), *The Culture of Japan as Seen Through Its Leisure*, Albany, NY: SUNY.

Omnés, R. 2002, *Quantum Philosophy*, Sangalli, A. (tr.), Woodstock (Oxford): Princeton University Press.

Ord, T. 2008, 'How to be a Consequentialist About Everything', presented at *The International Society for Utilitarian Studies*, Tenth Conference, University of California.

Parfit, D. 2017, *On What Matters* Vol. 3, Oxford: Oxford University Press.

Phillips, D. Z. 1976, 'Infinite Approximation', *Journal of the American Academy of Religion*, vol. 44, no. 3, pp. 477–487.

Phoenix, L. E. and Walter, L. (eds.). 2009, *Critical Food Issues: Problems and State-of-the-Art Solutions Worldwide*, Oxford: ABC-CLIO.

Plato. 1997, 'Protagoras', Lombardo, S. and Bell, K. (trs.), in Cooper, J. M. (ed.), *Plato: Complete Works*, Cambridge: Hackett.

————. 1994, 'Meno', in Day, J. M. (tr./ed.), *Plato's Meno in Focus*, London: Routledge, pp. 35–72.

Plato. 1921, *Theaetetus*, Fowler, H. N. (tr.), London: Harvard University Press.

————. 1966, 'Apology', in Fowler, H. N. (tr.), *Plato: Euthyphro, Apology, Crito, Phaedo, Phaedrus*, London: William Heinemann.

Qingyuan, X. 2000, Watts, A. (tr.), in Minford, J. and Lau, J. S. M. (eds.), *Classical Chinese Literature*, New York, NY: Columbia University Press, p. 975.

Ramachandran, V. S. and Hubbard, E. M. 2003, 'Hearing Colours, Tasting Shapes', *Scientific American*, vol. 288, no. 5, pp. 42–49.

Ramsey, I. T. 1957, *Religious Language: An Empirical Placing of Theological Phrases*, London: SCM Press.

Regan, T. 1983, *The Case for Animal Rights*, London: University of California Press, 2004.

Ricoeur, P. 1983, *Time and Narrative*, Vol. 1, McLaughlin, K. and Pellauer, D. (tr.), London: Chicago University Press, 1990.

Robertson, D. 2010, *The Philosophy of Cognitive Behavioural Therapy*, London: Karnac.

Roochnik, D. 2004, *Retrieving the Ancients*, Oxford: Blackwell.

Ross, W. D. 1930, *The Right and The Good*, Oxford: Oxford, University Press, 2002.

Rowlands, M. 2012, *Can Animals Be Moral?* Oxford, Oxford University Press.

————. 2013, *Animal Rights: All That Matters*, London: Hodder and Stoughton.

Russell, B. 1945, *A History of Western Philosophy*, London: Unwin, 1948.

Ryan, S. 1999, 'What Is Wisdom?' *Philosophical Studies: An International Journal for Philosophy in the Analytic Tradition*, vol. 93, no. 2, pp. 119–139.

Sanderson, R. B. and Pugliese, M. A. 2012, *Beyond Naïveté: Ethics, Economics, and Values*, Lanham, MD: University Press of America.

Schacht, R. 1976, 'Alienation: The Is-Ought Gap and Two Sorts of Discord', in Geyer, R. F. and Schweitzer, D. R. (eds.), *Theories of Alienation: Critical Perspectives in Philosophy and the Social Sciences*, Leiden: Springer, pp. 133–150.

Schweitzer, A. 1923, *Civilisation and Ethics*, Naish, J. (tr.), London: A and C Black.

————. 1951, *Letters, 1905–1965*, Neugroschel, J. (tr.), Bahr, H. W. (ed.), New York, NY: Macmillan, 1992.

Seymour, J. 1976, *The New Complete Book of Self-Sufficiency*, London: Dorling Kindersley, 2009.

Shakespeare, W. 1973, 'Hamlet: Prince of Denmark', in *The Complete Works of William Shakespeare*, London: Rex.

Sharzer, G. 2012, *No Local: Why Small Scale Alternatives Won't Change the World*, Alresford: Zero Books.

Siedentop, L. 2014, *Inventing the Individual: The Origins of Western Liberalism*, Cambridge, MA: Harvard University Press.

Singer, P. 2015, *The Most Good You Can Do: How Effective Altruism Is Changing Ideas About Living Ethically*, London: Yale University Press.

_____. 2006, 'Peter Singer: An Interview', *Satya*.

_____. 1975, *Animal Liberation: A New Ethics for Our Treatment of Animals*, New York, NY: Random House.

_____. 1979, *Practical Ethics*, Cambridge: Cambridge University Press, 1994.

_____. 1997, 'The Drowning Child and the Expanding Circle', in *The New Internationalist*.

_____. 2006, 'Peter Singer: An Interview', *Satya*.

Snowdon, P. F. 2014, *Persons, Animals, Ourselves*, Oxford: Oxford University Press.

Spaemann, R. 2006, *Persons: The Difference Between 'Someone' and 'Something'*, O'Donovan, O. (tr.), Oxford: Oxford University Press.

Stacey, J. 1997, *Teratologies: A Cultural Study of Cancer*, London: Routledge.

Stevens, W. 1967, 'Sunday Morning', in Stevens, W. (ed.), *Selected Poems*, London: Faber and Faber.

Strawson, G. 2004, 'Against Narrativity', in Ratio (new series), Vol. 17.

Strawson, P 1962, 'Freedom and Resentment', in Fischer, J. M. and Ravizza, M. (eds.), *Perspectives on Moral Responsibility*, London: Cornell University Press, 1993, pp. 45–66.

Taliaferro, C. 2001, 'The Virtues of Embodiment', *Philosophy*, vol. 76, no. 295, pp. 111–125.

Taylor, L. 2008, *A Taste for Gardening: Classed and Gendered Practices*, Oxford: Routledge.

Telfer, E. 1989–1990, 'The Unity of the Moral Virtues in Aristotle's "Nicomachean Ethics"', *Proceedings of the Aristotelian Society*, New Series, vol. 90, pp. 35–48.

Uebel, T. E. 1996, 'Neurath's Program for Naturalistic Epistemology', in Sarkar, S. (ed.), *Science and Philosophy in the Twentieth Century*, Harvard, MA: Harvard University Press.

Virgil. 1998, *Aeneid*, Day Lewis, C. (tr.), Oxford: Oxford University Press.

Vogel Carey, T. 2013, 'Consilience', *Philosophy Now*, vol. 95, pp. 25–27.

de Waal, F. 2001, *The Ape and the Sushi Master*, London: Penguin.

Waterfield, R. (tr.). 2000, *The First Philosophers*, Oxford: Oxford University Press.

Weil, S. 1943, *The Need for Roots: Prelude to a Declaration of Duties Towards Mankind*, Wills, A. (tr.), London: Routledge.

_____. 1941, 'Prerequisite to Dignity of Labour', in Miles, S. (ed.), *Simone Weil: An Anthology*, London: Virago Press, 1986.

Wharton, D. 2008, 'Wharton, David. "Sunt Lacrimae Rerum: An Exploration in Meaning"', *The Classical Journal*, vol. 103, no. 3, pp. 259–279.

White, N. P. 1994, 'Inquiry', in Day, J. M. (ed.), *Plato's Meno in Focus*, London: Routledge, pp. 152–171.

Whitehead, A. N. 1929, *Process and Reality*, New York, NY: First Free Press, 1985.

_____. 1981, 'The Importance of Free Will', Fischer, J. M. and Ravizza, M. (eds.), *Perspectives on Moral Responsibility*, London: Cornell University Press, 1993, pp. 101–118.

_____. 1982, 'Moral Saints', *The Journal of Philosophy*, vol. 79, no. 8, pp. 419–439.

Wiggins, D. 1988, 'Truth, Invention and the Meaning of Life', in Sayre-McCord, G. (ed.), *Essays on Moral Realism*, New York, NY: Cornell University Press.

Williams, B. 1985, *Ethics and the Limits of Philosophy*, Oxford: Routledge, 2006.

_____. 1981, 'Persons, Character and Morality', in Williams, B. (ed.), *Moral Luck*, Cambridge: Cambridge University Press.

Williams, B. and Smart, J. J. C. 1973, *Utilitarianism: For and Against*, Cambridge: Cambridge University Press.

Williams, R. 2014, *The Edge of Words*, London: Bloomsbury.

_____. 2012, 'Building Bridges in Istanbul', in Marshall, D. (ed.), *Science and Religion: Christian and Muslim Perspectives*, Washington, DC: Georgetown University Press.

Wilson, E. O. 1998, *Consilience*, New York, NY: Random House.

Winch, P. 1958, *The Idea of a Social Science and Its Relation to Philosophy*, Oxford: Routledge, 2008.

_____. 1959–1960, 'Nature and Convention', *Proceedings of the Aristotelian Society*, New Series, vol. 60, pp. 231–252.

Wittgenstein, L. 1969, *On Certainty*, Paul, D. and Anscombe, G. E. M. (tr.), Oxford: Blackwell, 1979.

_____. 1921, *Tractatus Logico-Philosophicus*, Pears, D. F. and McGuinness, B. F. (tr.), London: Routledge, 1961.

_____. 1929, 'A Lecture on Ethics', in *The Philosophical Review*, vol. 74, no. 1, 1965, pp. 3–12.

_____. 1940, *Culture and Value*, Winch, P. (tr.), von Wright, G. H. (ed.), London: University of Chicago Press, 1984.

_____. 1953, *Philosophical Investigations*, Anscombe, G. E. M. (tr.), Oxford: Blackwell, 2001.

Wolf, S. 2015, *The Variety of Values: Essays on Morality, Meaning and Love*, Oxford: Oxford University Press.

Zarefsky, D. 2014, *Rhetorical Perspectives on Argumentation*, London: Springer.

Zimmer, C. 2015, *Planet of Viruses – Second Edition*, London: University of Chicago Press.

Index

Printed in the United States
by Baker & Taylor Publisher Services